William Fraser Rae

Austrian health resorts throughout the year

Second Edition

William Fraser Rae

Austrian health resorts throughout the year
Second Edition

ISBN/EAN: 9783744744607

Printed in Europe, USA, Canada, Australia, Japan

Cover: Foto ©ninafisch / pixelio.de

More available books at **www.hansebooks.com**

AUSTRIAN HEALTH RESORTS

THROUGHOUT THE YEAR

BY

W. FRASER RAE

REPRINTED, BY PERMISSION, FROM

The Times

SECOND AND ENLARGED EDITION

LONDON: CHAPMAN AND HALL
LIMITED
1889

THIS WORK IS DEDICATED

TO

Dr. B. London, of Carlsbad,

FROM WHOM THE AUTHOR HAS RECEIVED MUCH KINDNESS AND
GOOD ADVICE.

PREFACE TO THE SECOND EDITION.

CHAPTERS XIV. and XV. in this Edition have been added in place of the Chapter in the first on "The Bitter Waters of Hungary." Thus the present Edition of this book treats exclusively of noteworthy places in the Empire of Austria, many of which are seldom visited by Englishmen or Americans, and are scarcely known to them even by repute. Yet each deserves to be visited by those who journey in quest of health or variety. An invalid requiring a course of mineral waters may go to Carlsbad, Franzensbad, Marienbad, or some other Austrian Health Resort in the spring, summer, or autumn; another, to whom the grape "cure" is prescribed, may visit Vöslau or Meran in the autumn; the invalid who desires sea bathing in perfection can enjoy it for several months out of the twelve at Abbazia; while any one who is in quest of a mild and pleasant winter climate may find it at Meran, or Arco, Abbazia, or Gorizia. I may add, with confidence and perfect truth, that the geniality of the people lends an additional charm to all the Health Resorts in the Empire of Austria.

NOTE.—In the first paragraph of the Introduction, "Tepitz" should read Teplitz, and in the third, "Rocegno" should read Roncegno.

INTRODUCTION.

MUCH of the first chapter in this work appeared in an article on Carlsbad which was published in *The Nineteenth Century* for November, 1884, and in another in *The Times* for the 22nd of August, 1885. Having revisited Carlsbad since these articles appeared, I have embodied the results of my further experience in that chapter. It is so much changed, as well as enlarged, as to be new in form, though not in subject. In it, as in the chapters treating of Franzensbad and Marienbad, details are set forth concerning Goethe's visits which are not to be found in the late G. H. Lewes's "Life" of that extraordinary man. The particulars given with regard to Peter the Great's sojourn at Carlsbad and Tepitz are not to be met with in the recent and elaborate work on him from the pen of Mr. Eugene Schuyler.

The chapter on Königswart is new, and many other chapters are greatly altered and enlarged. I have revisited several of the places described since first writing about them, and it was fitting that I should treat them in this work from the point of view from which I last saw them. Moreover, the articles written for the reader who has not more than a day in which to peruse them ought to be cast in a somewhat different mould when they are prepared for publication in book form.

This book is not intended to come into competition with preceding ones on Health Resorts in Austria and Hungary. Most of those works which enjoy the patronage and merit the admiration of the public have been compiled by medical men, and they contain information of a purely professional kind, whilst they may be lacking in other information which, though less technical, is better adapted to please and instruct the general reader—a personage more indolent than any reviewer, and one who likes the path to be made very smooth. To such a reader the most careful and trustworthy analysis of a mineral water may not convey many clear ideas. Probably he or she does not care to peruse the lists of ingredients in a mineral spring. Even the reader who has a smattering of chemical knowledge may be unable to understand scientific terminology which is often foreign in character, and which is sometimes old-fashioned and obsolete. In one case only have I departed from my rule not to fill pages with tables of analyses, which would not be understood by ordinary readers, and which might be deemed surplusage by others. The exception is the analysis of the water which is found at Rocegno. In none of the English works which I have consulted is any account given of this notable arsenical-ferruginous water. In reproducing an analysis of it I may render a service to those who are curious to have these particulars and may not know where to find them.

Whilst purposely omitting details which might not have any interest outside of a limited circle of possible readers, I have endeavoured to furnish those which may attract and instruct the reader who intends to visit the Health Resorts named in this work, and the readers who may wish to know something about them without leaving home. It is for the benefit of the latter that not only are the places described as they now are, but that historical facts are given concerning their rise and progress. For instance, no account is given in any English work, so far as I know, of the valley of Gastein in the days when it was the El Dorado of Europe, and when it was as much valued as a place rich in the precious metals as California and Australia are at the present day. Moreover, none of the writers about it have thought fit to reproduce some interesting facts which the famous William von Humboldt has left on record of his personal experiences there sixty years ago. Some professional men may consider particulars such as these unworthy of their notice. Unless I greatly err, the reading public will accept them with gratitude.

Whilst several of the places described in this work are well known by name, others are not more familiar to the ordinary reader than the chief places of note in the heart of Central Africa or on the shores of Hudson Bay. For my own part, I was surprised to find in the Austrian Tyrol three Health Resorts of which the names had seldom appeared in an English book, yet which were quite as noteworthy as some of the most frequented watering-places in the Pyrenees, and the most fashionable spots on the Riviera. I have set forth their attractions with entire impartiality, yet not without a feeling of regret that these beautiful places will some day be overcrowded and will then be less enjoyable.

Amongst the many mineral springs in Austria and Hungary there may be several quite as noteworthy as those which are described in this work. I have purposely chosen a few which, though in high repute for many years, and even for centuries, are not yet familiar to all the English and American seekers after pleasant and health-restoring places of sojourn. There was a time in the history of the oldest spring when its virtues were supposed to be almost miraculous. No one could tell why those who drank or bathed in it were healed of their infirmities. The mystery is not yet wholly removed; yet the knowledge of every spring has been increased an hundredfold. The analytic chemist can determine their contents, and the skilled physician now can form an approximate guess as to the way in which the waters act, and as to the best way in which they should be used. I do not believe that the veil has been entirely withdrawn, or that the spirit of the spring has been disclosed to full view. In the days of antiquity a god was believed to preside over every spring. Sir Walter Scott may have had such a notion in his mind when he depicted, with less than his usual success, the White Lady of Avenel in "The Monastery." He gave expression to a similar view when he made Mrs. Meg Dods say, in another novel, that the medicinal virtue of St. Ronan's Well was due to the Saint having ducked the Devil in it and thereby imparted a sulphurous character to the water. The Spanish adventurers who first explored the New World had a firm expectation of finding not only precious metals there, but a Fountain of Youth more precious still. When Juan Ponce de Leon headed an expedition to Florida, he and his companions eagerly drank of every spring of living water, in the hope that they might gain perpetual youth. They were less fortunate than the old Indian of whom Peter Martyr writes that the Indian, being "grievously oppressed with old age, moved with the fame of that fountain, and allured by the love longer of life, went from his native island unto the country of Florida to drink of the desired fountain . . . and having well drunk and washed himself for many days with the appointed remedies, by them who kept the bath, he is reported to have brought home a manly strength, and to have used all manly exercises, and that he married again and begat children."

Though science has disclosed the chief secrets of mineral springs, there are yet some hidden mysteries to be divulged. I have shown in the chapter on Gastein how divergent are the views taken of the reasons why the mineral water there should be so powerful in its action. I have read many tales about the effects of other mineral springs which are hardly less strange than the fabulous tale about the old Indian in Florida. Instead, however, of filling pages with these stories of natural magic, I have striven to ascertain and set forth actual facts; and in not a few cases the facts are nearly as extraordinary as any fictions.

Nothing is more striking at the principal Austrian Health Resorts than the completeness of the arrangements for turning the waters to the best account. Indeed, many of the cures are due in part to the way in which the water is employed, and to the skill and experience of the physicians under whose direction patients follow the treatment. In early days, as I have shown by the history of Franzensbad and Marienbad, the seeker after health had to suffer much discomfort at a mineral spring; but the drawbacks were speedily removed, and the places which had been abodes of misery were transformed into temples of luxury. Few of the English Health Resorts are arranged with equal regard for the fancies and conveniences of invalids. The neglect from which many suffer is explainable on this ground. Some springs on the Continent are not of greater intrinsic value than that of Epsom, which has long fallen into disrepute. No efforts were ever made to render a sojourn at it attractive; and interesting evidence on this head is to be found in the "Letters" which were written by Dorothy Osborne, between 1652 and 1654, to Sir William Temple, whose wife she afterwards became, and which have recently been published under the editorship of Mr. E. A. Parry. Both of them went to Epsom for what Germans call "the cure." Dorothy thus commented on a letter in which Sir William narrated his experience:

"However, I cannot but wish you had stayed longer at Epsom and drunk the waters with more order though in a less proportion. But did you drink them immediately from the well? I remember I was forbid it, and methought with a good deal of reason, for (especially at this time of year) the well is so low, and there is such a multitude to be served out on't, that you can hardly get any but what is thick and troubled; and I have marked that when it stood all night (for that was my direction) the bottom of the vessel it stood in would be covered an inch thick with white clay, which, sure, has no great virtue in't, and is not very pleasant to drink."

Whilst the Health Resorts on the Continent are

more highly prized than those in England, and are systematically planned to induce the sick to visit them, they owe much to the medical men who make a study of balneology and who are specially qualified for giving sound advice on the spot. I have collected many German books and pamphlets treating of the places I visited, and I have extracted from them the salient facts. The painstaking character and the profundity of German writers are proverbial. Medical men in Germany and Austria are as averse as German philosophers from taking anything for granted; and sometimes they attach an importance to simple things which would not be shown in a professional work written in English. For instance, it is superfluous to warn a patient against going out of doors when the weather is bad, to advise him to carry an umbrella when it looks like rain, or to say that it is prudent to try the temperature of a bath with the finger or toe instead of rashly plunging in at the risk of being scalded.

I have given my authorities for any purely medical matter quoted; but the reader who desires medical details rather than general information is referred to works by members of the medical profession. This work does not profess to be a "Guide:" there are plenty of excellent guide-books in existence. Its purpose is to be a supplement to the technical books on Health Resorts, and to the books in which the traveller learns all about roads, rails, and hotels, how to reach a particular place, where to live and what to see there, and how to leave it.

During the publication of the articles upon which this book is based, a short article appeared in *The Lancet* which sets forth their scope in better terms than any which I could employ. In the belief that it will interest many readers and commend this book to their notice, I subjoin it: "*The Times* of June 22nd began publishing a series of articles 'from a correspondent,' on Austrian Health Resorts, which cannot fail to be of much interest to many who are contemplating an autumnal holiday to some Continental inland watering-place. The gouty, the rheumatic, the dyspeptic, and the over-wrought find in such a change relief and invigoration, which strictly medicinal treatment at home often fails to accomplish. It is not sufficient for such persons that their change should have a directly medical object, and be confined to drinking this or that natural mineral water, though this may form a very important element for the relief of their discomfort. But the air, scenery, elevation above sea level, as well as amusements and novel experiences of life, with facilities for travelling, are matters needing careful preliminary consideration, both by the doctor and the patient. The medical adviser has much difficulty in selecting the kind of place that is likely to be beneficial as well as agreeable to his patient. A large number of persons who go to Continental watering-places need the one as much as the other. Numbers of persons can be equally well-treated, medicinally, at any one of three or four places, though in some instances, no doubt, a particular place is best suited to a particular case; and this is a matter which medical opinion can best settle. But in other instances, where the appurtenances of medical treatment have to be considered, the patient may fairly have a voice in the selection, and he could scarcely do better than read the articles referred to in order to fit himself to exercise a right judgment in this respect; nor are the articles without their value to medical men."

CONTENTS.

	PAGE
CHAPTER I.—CARLSBAD	1
Fables about the "Sprudel"	3
Notable Visitors	5
Heroic Treatment	7
The Preliminary Ordeal	9
A Bold Innovator	11
Nature of the Treatment	13
The Daily Round	15
What to Eat and Drink	17
"Medical Vampires"	19
"Carry an Umbrella"	21
Goethe at Carlsbad	23
His Fourth Visit	25
Public Gaming Tables	27
An Eccentric Duke	29
A Pleasant Surprise	31
Peter the Great	33
An Imperial Mason	35
Leibnitz and the Czar	37

CHAPTER I.—CARLSBAD (continued).

	PAGE
Picturesque Walks	39
Frequenters of the Springs	41
Magnates and Millionaires	43
Patients and Doctors	45
Baths and Waters	47
The Emperor's Birthday	49
The Queen of Watering Places	51

CHAPTER II.—GIESSHÜBL-PUCHSTEIN. 52

A Pleasant Beverage	53
King Otto's Spring	55
Natural Charms	57
Increasing Demand	59
Pretty and Picturesque	61

CHAPTER III.—FRANZENSBAD. 62

A Ladies' Bath	63
A Petticoat Riot	65
Springs and Baths	67
Despotic Doctors	69
The Bill of Fare	71
Early to Bed	73
Impatience Improper	75
An Extinct Volcano	77
The Moor at Soos	79
Palæontological Treasures	81
Frederick the Great Cured	83
An Historical Event	85

CONTENTS.

	PAGE
CHAPTER IV.—MARIENBAD	86
"Very Thick Ladies"	87
An Unexpected Discovery	89
Rash Water-drinkers	91
Goethe's First Visit	93
In a Moor-bath	95
Effect of a Gas-bath	97
Character of the Springs	99
A Family Watering-place	101
A Bill of Fare	103
Sleeping and Starving	105
Churches and Amusements	107
A Wonderful Water	109
CHAPTER V.—TEPLITZ	110
Illustrious Visitors	111
A Catastrophe	113
The Springs Rediscovered	115
Bathing or Shampooing?	117
Milk, Water, and Beer	119
Going on Pilgrimage	121
Battles and Monuments	123
An Exceptional Spring	125
CHAPTER VI.—KÖNIGSWART	126
Invigorating Waters	127
A Sanatorium	129

CONTENTS.

CHAPTER VI.—KÖNIGSWART (continued).

	PAGE
A Romantic Career	131
Odds and Ends	133
The Bohemian Legislature	135
Home Rule in Bohemia	137
Lucrative Patriotism	139
German Demands	141
Mr. Freeman's Comments	143

CHAPTER VII.—BADEN AND VÖSLAU . . . 145

The Two Badens	147
A Roman Bath	149
Fire and Pestilence	151
Unadulterated Wine	153
A Trying Water	155
Good Advice	157
A Choice of Cures	159
A Blot on the Landscape	161

CHAPTER VIII.—ISCHL . . . 163

Brine Baths and Whey	165
Viennese Journalists	167
Daughters of Luxury	169
Russian Baths	171
Butter-milk Cure	173
The Curhaus	175
Natural Attractions	177

CONTENTS.

	PAGE
CHAPTER IX.—GASTEIN	179
Ancient Gold-mining	181
Persecuted Protestants	183
Doctors and Hotels	185
The Valley	187
The Waterfall	189
Indifferent Waters	191
Effect of Mineral Water	193
Revivifying Flowers	195
Idle Hands	197
Miraculous Water	199
Times and Seasons	201
CHAPTER X.—MERAN	203
The Grape Cure	205
A Light Diet	207
A Grape Problem	209
The Pleasantest "Cure"	211
An Imperial Visitor	213
A Windless Valley	215
Testimony of the Rocks	217
Winter Amusements	219
CHAPTER XI.—RONCEGNO	221
Out of the Beaten Track	223
A Golden-yellow Liquid	225
A Potent Medicine	227

CHAPTER XI.—RONCEGNO (*continued*).

	PAGE
Rules and Regulations	229
How and When to Bathe	231
Character of the Water	233
Growing Popular	235
The Tesino Valley	237
Scenery and Climate	239

CHAPTER XII.—LEVICO

	241
Points of Interest	243
A Popular Poison	245
Arsenical Water	247
The Doctor's Fee	249
Bathing Under Difficulties	251
Superfluous Advice	253
International Medicine	255
"Care Hinders Cure"	257

CHAPTER XIII.—ARCO

	258
The Beauties of Nature	259
A Medical Critic	261
Weather in Winter	263
The Dust Plague	265
The Golden Mean	267
The Terrain Cure	269
Rival Health Resorts	271
The Bane of Popularity	273
An Austrian Paradise	275

CONTENTS.

	PAGE
CHAPTER XIV.—ABBAZIA.	276
A Benedictine Abbey.	277
A Predestined Health Resort	279
Royal and Titled Visitors	281
Nice in Summer.	283
The Fiume Gulf.	285
Winter Temperature.	287
Water and Gas.	289
Pestiferous Odours	291
Systematic Sea Bathing	293
Walks and Excursions	295
CHAPTER XV.—GORIZIA	297
Beginning of the City.	299
The Austrian Nice	301
Temperature in Winter	303
Character of the Climate	305
A Clean City	307
Amusements	309
Hotels and Villas.	311
Provisions and Wine	313
Castagnavizza	315
A Beautiful Prospect.	317

AUSTRIAN HEALTH RESORTS.

CHAPTER I.

CARLSBAD.

BOHEMIA is characterised at the heading to the third scene in the third act of *The Winter's Tale* as "a desert country near the sea." Shakespeare is held to have displayed inexcusable ignorance in making Antigonus land upon the Bohemian sea-coast, and the plea of poetic licence has not availed to save him from censure. Yet an excuse might be urged for his blunder, which, though not conclusive, is yet quite as good as the excuses proffered by enthusiastic commentators in extenuation of other blunders in his plays.

In Shakespeare's day Bohemia was famed for its watering-places, and he may have supposed that, where a watering-place existed, the sea was not very far off. Whether he were misled by something which he had heard and misunderstood, or whether, as is more probable, he simply drew upon his imagination for his localities, it is certain that the fame of one Bohemian watering-place had spread far and wide long before Shakespeare was born. This was Carlsbad, a place which Herr Karl Böttcher likens to "a full-blown rose placed upon Austria's bosom to beautify and adorn it."

Geologists affirm that the healing waters of Carlsbad have issued from the ground since a time of which the rocks are the only record. How long these waters have been turned to medicinal account cannot be determined with precision; but it is beyond doubt that they have been highly valued as medicines during six centuries. Most of the mineral springs which are still in high repute were discovered and used by the Romans, who seem to have had as keen eyes for mineral waters as the North American Indians. Yet the Carlsbad waters apparently escaped the notice of those conquerors of the world to whom mineral water was only less dear than universal dominion. A fable was long accepted as the true explanation of the discovery of these waters. It ran to the effect that, on the 23rd of June, 1370, the Emperor Charles the Fourth was hunting the stag near the valley in which Carlsbad now stands. The animal pursued by the hunters leapt from the high ground into this valley, whither the hounds followed. When one of the hunters descended to the bottom of the valley, he saw the hounds struggling for their lives in a huge natural cauldron of seething water. The "Sprudel," the principal spring at Carlsbad, now rises from this spot in the form of a small geyser, the temperature being 165° Fahrenheit.

As the water is so hot, the glasses are filled by being placed in a small holder at the end of a long pole. This is a practical exemplification of the Scottish saying: "When you sup with the Devil you must have a long spoon." Perhaps I may here explain that those who now go to Carlsbad in the belief that the Sprudel water contains gold will be disappointed. A paragraph to the effect that gold has been discovered in it has gone the round of the English and American papers. No contradiction has appeared in them, yet there is no truth in the statement. It originated in the columns of the *Karlsbader Zeitung*, which appears on Sunday, and this year the 1st of April fell on a Sunday. What the Carlsbad journalist meant as a joke has been accepted as a fact. There are many mineral ingredients in the Sprudel water, but gold is not one of them.

The oldest statement about the Sprudel is no more authentic than the latest. What militates against the allegation of the Emperor Charles the Fourth having been the first discoverer of the "Sprudel," either through the intermediary of a stag or a dog, or in his own person, is the undoubted circumstance of the spring being known to King John, his father. It is possible that the Emperor bathed in it, and that the place was named after him.

King John and the Emperor Charles the Fourth were the first of many crowned heads who have visited Carlsbad as patients. Out of the long list the names may be cited of Frederick the First of Prussia; Peter the Great; Augustus the First of Poland; the Emperor Charles the Sixth; the Empress Maria Ludovika; a king of Saxony; the Emperor Francis the Second and his daughter, the Empress Maria Louisa, the second wife of Bonaparte; Frederick William the Third of Prussia; and his successor William, the First German Emperor. The lovely but most unfortunate Empress Eugénie has visited Carlsbad more than once, deriving much benefit from the waters. The names of some other visitors will be cherished with warm affection long after those of many royal personages are forgotten. Amongst them are Sebastian Bach and Beethoven; Catalini, Sontag, and Paganini; Gellert, Fichte, and Schelling; Herder, Schiller, and Goethe; Körner, Auerbach, Strauss, and Tourgenieff; Chateaubriand and Gervinus. The third Duke of Wellington is one of the many notable English visitors at the present day. Prince Blücher visited Carlsbad after Waterloo, and Prince Bismarck before Sadowa. A story is told of Blücher that, after arriving and taking the waters, he exclaimed: "I always detested water-drinking, yet the Devil has brought me here to swallow water against my will."

The name of every visitor to Carlsbad is now printed and published. It was not till the year 1756 that a complete record of them was kept. In that year the visitors numbered 134; the number of those who now go thither between the months of May and October in each year does not fall short of 30,000, and it is sometimes in excess of these figures. The chief knowledge which we have of the way in which the waters were valued three or four centuries ago, is derived from a Latin ode written by Bohuslaw Lobkowitz, who died in 1510. He there writes that the waters merit all the praise which the Muse can bestow, that they are great natural marvels as well as most valuable medicinal products, that their use restores vigour to the body and limbs of the old, and revives the rosy bloom of health in the cheeks of the delicate maiden.

In the days when Bohuslaw Lobkowitz lived and praised the healing springs at Carlsbad, they were used for bathing and not for drinking; now they are chiefly valued for their effects when taken internally. Two centuries elapsed after they had become famous before medical men ordered their patients to drink them. During the period when bathing was the rule, the process was a serious one, judging from the account of it which was written in 1571 by Dr. Summers. The passage which is quoted in Dr. Hlawacek's elaborate work on Carlsbad is in a form of German that is nearly as obsolete as Chaucer's English. I may translate it as follows: "When it is desired to cause an eruption over the body and skin, the patient must bathe for ten or eleven hours daily, beginning with a few baths the first day, bathing for three hours in the morning and two in the afternoon, increasing the time by one, two, three, and more hours afterwards till the eruption has occurred. The water must not be so cold as to give the patient a chill, but should be tepid only, and not so warm as to induce perspiration when the eruption has broken out on the skin. When this eruption has taken place, the patient is to leave the bath, cover himself with wraps, and walk up and down in a moderately warm room; or, if this should be a labour to him, he is to lie down in bed so that the evil humours may have free course to the surface. After an hour or two he is to return to the bath, and remain an hour there, and then leave it, remaining in his room so that the evil humours may recommence to flow. Thereafter he is to return to the bath, remaining there for an hour, and this he is to do, so far as may be practicable, four or five times during two, three, or more days, till the flow of the evil humours has ceased. When this happens he is to bathe again, not in the water which caused the eruption, but in other and unused water. On the first day this water is not to be very warm, but should be cooled down, yet it should be warmer than the water which caused the eruption; afterwards he is to bathe for a longer time in warmer water till the skin is drawn together. When the patient begins to bathe in warm water, he is to do so four or five times a day, for fifteen or thirty minutes at a time, and, when he leaves the bath, he is to remain for an hour in a warm room. During the following days he is to prolong his stay in the bath from day to day."

When a patient was covered with painful boils he was pronounced in a fair way towards recovery. Few invalids and few maladies could long resist this heroic treatment, it was eminently a case of kill or cure; yet the cures seem to have predominated. Strong measures were in favour with our stalwart forefathers, and what might sap the energies of their more sensitive, if not degenerate descendants, appears to have given them fresh vigour and a renewed lease of life. Perhaps the skins of those who were never thoroughly washed, except immediately after birth and death, may have been tougher than those of the persons who, in our day, regularly wash their bodies as well as their faces. It is noteworthy that the original mode of treating disease in olden days at Carlsbad is the same as that which has always been in vogue amongst some North American Indians. These Indians never wash themselves till they are ill and find a hot spring, and then they remain in the water till they are parboiled and better.

Two centuries after invalids had been boiled and baked at Carlsbad, and either left it cured or remained there for ever, Dr. Payer, one of the resident physicians, introduced a new method of treatment. He wrote in a book published in 1520:—"I am of opinion that this water should be drunk. However, as it has been chiefly used for external and not for internal use, many persons will consider this a novel proposal." Dr. Payer was a contemporary of Paracelsus, who, though a regular medical practitioner, was regarded as a quack by many persons, because he had the audacity to prescribe mercury and opium to his patients. With as great rashness, Dr. Payer was denounced as a quack by his colleagues at

Carlsbad; they did not approve of such an innovation as advising the waters to be drunk as well as bathed in.

It is true that the patient who drank the Carlsbad mineral water in obedience to the advice of Dr. Payer had an ordeal to pass through which was hardly less trying than that of the patient who bathed in it till he was covered with boils. Whether one drank or bathed in mineral water, one was obliged in those days to undergo a severe course of physic. This was the rule in France as well as in Bohemia. Dr. John Macpherson has quoted a passage on this head in his admirable book on "The Baths and Wells of Europe." It is taken from a letter which Boileau sent to Racine describing his personal experience as a patient: "I have been purged and bled, and have not failed to comply with all the formalities required before commencing the use of the waters. The medicine which I have taken to-day has, as they pleasantly say, done me all the good in the world, for it has made me faint four or five times, and rendered me so weak that I can scarcely stand."

Up to the beginning of the eighteenth century it was common at Carlsbad to subject the patient to a preliminary course of violent purgatives. He or she was supposed to be suffering from repletion. After having been weakened by strong medicines, the patient was ordered to drink the mineral water for seven days, and to bathe in it for the following seven days, drinking and bathing for successive weeks till the patient was cured or a corpse.

At present it is not common to drink more than three glasses of the water, and the immediate effect is not more marked or unpleasant than when the like quantity of spring water is drunk. But early in the eighteenth century, and for many years later, intemperance in drinking mineral water was the rule. Dr. Hofmann, an estimable physician in his day, writing in 1705, says that no more than from fifteen to eighteen glasses should be taken the first day of the treatment, and that the patient should gradually increase the dose till the glasses emptied numbered forty. Dr. Tilling, who was a patient in 1756, records that he drank from fifty to sixty glasses of water in the course of two hours. Dr. Sangrado did not prescribe warm water in larger doses, and the puzzle is how the patients at Carlsbad in those days succeeded in carrying out the orders of the doctor. The natives of the Queen Charlotte Islands are in the habit of swallowing a bucket of sea water when they feel out of health; but they do not expect to retain the water long. In those days the patients at Carlsbad did not drink large quantities of water in order to make themselves sick. The explanation of their being able to drink so copiously without the water acting as an emetic, is the drinking of the water took place in a warm room, and that most of it passed off in perspiration. Indeed the patients were ordered to remain in a warm place so as to perspire the more freely.

In 1777, Dr. David Becher, a physician whose bust in bronze is now one of the ornaments of the large hall where the drinkers at the Sprudel walk in a semi-circle after drinking water, and whilst listening to the band, appeared as an innovator at Carlsbad, and was regarded and treated accordingly. Dr. Becher had the audacity to assert and maintain that the water should be drunk at the spring, instead of indoors. His views were first denounced and then accepted.

Besides upholding the propriety of going to the fountain-head for mineral water, Dr. Becher concluded that the quantity taken should be regulated in accordance with the effect which it was desired to produce. This now appears to be a commonplace; in Dr. Becher's day it was regarded as a paradox. Yet Dr. Becher prevailed; his system of treatment was eventually adopted by the colleagues who had thought it their duty to denounce it as preposterous. His wisdom was justified by its results. Year after year the rules which Dr. Becher had enjoined were enforced by physicians who wisely accepted his teaching. Yet the earlier habit of drinking too much water lasted longer than was justifiable on rational grounds. So late as 1834 the ordinary dose was from twelve to fifteen glasses; it is now from three to four. At a time when human beings were treated as if they were lower animals, it was common to subject the lower animals to a course of Carlsbad mineral water. The Mühlbrum was then set apart for the treatment of sick horses, dogs, and cattle. The same spring is now the one most frequented by invalids; but neither it nor any other is any longer used for the treatment of the lower creation.

Amongst the many notable changes in dealing with patients at Carlsbad, not the least instructive are those which affected vested interests. Most of the houses, wherein patients took up their abode, had a mineral spring on the premises. The proprietors of these houses considered it improper that any one who tenanted them should think of drinking or bathing in mineral water elsewhere. Much trouble was occasioned by the demands of those who preferred the ancient ways. So long as they walked, or rather compelled others to walk in them, they made much money. They objected to their gains being curtailed. However, an end was made to private enterprise of this sort, and no patient can now drink mineral water except that which is yielded by springs which are free to all strangers who have paid the tax imposed upon them. Some invalids may have suffered by this change; but the majority have been benefited. The municipality has become the sole proprietor of the Carlsbad mineral springs, and all the arrangements now made with regard to them are in the interests alike of the inhabitants and the visitors.

Few persons who have not sojourned at Carlsbad entertain correct notions as to the mode of life there. The opinion generally prevails that the unhappy patient is dosed with mineral water till he is reduced to a skeleton, and that to hasten the cure, which has the character of a killing one, the patient is put on starvation diet. It is true, as I have already shown, that formerly the course of treatment, whether the water were applied in the form of baths or employed for drinking, had a purgatorial tendency. It is equally true that the rules with respect to diet were strict to the verge of absurdity.

Many persons go to Carlsbad because they have lived too well and grown too stout. That abstinence from certain kinds of food and liquids should be enjoined in the cases of such persons seems perfectly proper. Yet those who cannot eat much or digest anything with ease are also told that they must avoid particular articles of diet. They are warned against drinking beer or eating butter and cheese, salad, uncooked fruit and ices; and stories are current about the sad fate of those who have indulged in forbidden dainties. Some of these stories are as horrible and untrue as the ghost stories with which superstitious nurses frighten naughty children. One of them is to the effect that an Englishman, after having drunk a glass of Sprudel water, ate two cherries and died. Other persons are said to have endangered their lives by eating a little butter and drinking a glass of beer whilst undergoing the treatment.

In diet, as in the mode of taking the waters, the physicians at Carlsbad have held varying and sometimes contradictory opinions. Thus, whilst butter is now amongst the articles which are not *Curgemäss*, that is not in accord with the "cure," it was once ordered to be eaten. A physician writing in 1710 said it was the proper thing, at the end of each meal, to eat a quantity of fresh butter, over which carraway seeds were strewed. The same writer advised patients to eat roast meat at their early dinner, boiled meat at their early supper, and to drink well-fermented beer. Whilst there can be no doubt that fixed rules as regards diet have their advantages, it is certain that the value of the rules largely depends on their application to individual cases. Patients from all parts of the world visit Carlsbad. In Russia, Italy,

France, England, Germany, America, and other countries, the mode of living differs, and what would be considered excess in one country might really be moderation in another. To disregard this self-evident consideration is as foolish as the conduct of the English physician of note in the last century who based his treatment upon the supposition that most diseases had their origin in the itch, and that few persons had escaped that loathsome malady. The truth is, there are few things that may not be eaten with impunity during a course of Carlsbad waters, provided moderation be practised, and provided also that the patient is not suffering from a disease which compels abstinence from these articles of food at all times.

Dr. Hlawacek, who practised as a physician at Carlsbad during forty years, and whose work, as I have already said, is the most comprehensive one concerning that place, lays down the following rules with regard to regimen.

According to him, patients are to begin the day by rising not later than six, and walking to the springs. After drinking, at intervals of fifteen minutes, three glasses of the particular water prescribed, and taking gentle exercise for an hour after the last glass, they may breakfast. For breakfast Dr. Hlawacek recommends from one to two cups of coffee with milk, chocolate or cocoa, accompanied by two small rolls, which he is careful to add will cost two kreutzers, or less than a penny each. It may be noted in passing that the custom prevails in Carlsbad of the patients going to baker's shops and buying the rolls or rusks which they eat at breakfast or supper, and carrying them to the *café* or restaurant where the rest of the meal is provided.

The dinner hour at Carlsbad is between twelve and two o'clock. At dinner three courses are allowed; these consist of soup, meat, and a dish of vegetables, and those who prefer it may substitute some cooked fruit or a light pudding for the vegetables. Dr. Hlawacek objects to patients frequenting a *table d'hôte*, on the ground that they may be tempted to over-eat themselves. His fears in this matter are ill-founded, as no *table d'hôte* is to be found in any Carlsbad hotel. He is emphatic in stating that the soup should be very plain and devoid of fat, meaning by this, no doubt, that it should be watery and tasteless. Whatever the soup may have been in his days, it is now very good, and far better than is provided in the majority of French restaurants. The kinds of meat which he sanctions are tender beef, veal, lamb, or mutton; unfortunately, it is easier to procure good soup than good and tender meat in Carlsbad, much of the meat having the flavour and toughness of cooked string. But the patient may eat fowls or game, with the exception of the skin—an exception with which no civilised person will quarrel; and, happily, the Bohemian fowls and game are excellent. Hare and venison are classed amongst the prohibited articles of diet, whilst such fish as trout, pike, and carp are pronounced *Curgemäss*, the skin being always excepted. Why it should be thought needful to forbid the eating of the skin of fish or fowl is a puzzle to me: it would be as sensible to forbid the eating of the bones. The vegetables which are allowed include spinach, carrots, cauliflower, green peas, French beans, asparagus, and mashed potatoes. When cooked, such fruits as cherries, plums, and apricots are permitted; but all pastry is condemned, especially the sweet wafer biscuits which are known in Carlsbad as *Oblaten*, and which have been imitated in England under the name of Carlsbad wafers. As an exception, Dr. Hlawacek sometimes permits such raw fruits to be eaten as strawberries, grapes, and oranges. He holds that white bread should be chosen in preference to black, a preference which is in entire accord with French and English taste, and he maintains that stale bread is more digestible than newly baked bread, an opinion which many people share. Water he pronounces the best beverage, yet he does not disapprove of Austrian, Hungarian, French, or German wines being taken in quantities not exceeding half a bottle daily. Since he lived and wrote, it has become the rule for all who drink water only, or who mix water with wine, to select for the purpose the delicious sparkling table water which is known as Giesshübler, and which comes from Giesshübl-Puchstein, a watering-place about seven miles distant.

Austrians and Germans are in the habit of taking a very light repast called *Vesperbrod*, which corresponds to the English five o'clock tea. Coffee with cream is said by Dr. Hlawacek to be the favourite drink at this time, and a roll is generally eaten. He disapproves of the coffee, the cream, and the roll, and he advises sensible persons to take instead of them the still lighter refreshment of aërated water. He affirms that the water will do them as much good as the coffee, cream, and roll will do them harm. Certainly it will not produce a sensation of repletion.

Supper is a simple meal, consisting of a little soup, a roll, and some stewed fruit, or two soft-boiled eggs. Those who require something more substantial are permitted to eat a slice of raw ham, a permission upon which American and English patients will decline to act. The patients are advised to drink water at supper; but those who are addicted to tea-drinking are allowed to take tea, provided it be tepid and very weak, as it usually is at Carlsbad. The conscientious patients, who wish to give the mineral water the best chance of working a complete cure, are advised to go to bed fasting. Those who are ordered to bathe in as well as to drink the waters, take baths between breakfast and dinner every other day. All spare time between meals is to be occupied in taking exercise in the open air. After a well-spent day, during which obedient patients have displayed as great self-denial and have covered as much ground as if they were in training for a walking match, and have fared like anchorites, they go to bed between nine and ten o'clock, there to rest their weary limbs and dream of dining with Lucullus.

Dr. Hlawacek admits that patients at Carlsbad require a mental as well as a physical form of treatment. He wisely thinks that if they do not keep up their spirits, they cannot get up their strength. He enjoins the necessity of their throwing off all worldly cares, and living for their health alone, without thinking too much about it; and, whilst he considers it fitting that they should receive frequent letters from home, he objects to their tiring themselves by writing at length in return. He warns them against "the medical vampires" who get into conversation with patients, make them dissatisfied with their medical advisers, and give them bad advice. He recommends patients to confine their reading to light literature and especially to newspapers, which he accounts the lightest of all reading. If they will play at cards, they must not play for high stakes, or for several hours at a time. He thinks that they would do better to play at billiards, and that they would do better still if they took walks and enjoyed the natural beauties which abound in the neighbourhood.

Not till the labours of drinking mineral water, or bathing in it, and taking the enjoined amount of physical exercise are ended, does Dr. Hlawacek approve of patients going to sleep. However drowsy they may feel during the day, they must resist the temptation to sleep, and must strive to keep their eyes open by bathing their faces in cold water or moistening them with eau-de-cologne. Those who cannot sleep at night, may indulge in a nap on the sofa before dinner; but they do so at their peril, as it is pronounced dangerous to make a practice of succumbing by day to this weakness of the flesh. If they have strictly followed the advice given to them by Dr. Hlawacek and some of his successors, they will go to bed famished and weary, and regard their couch as the best of all places, and sleep as a true comforter.

In addition to telling patients what to eat, drink, and avoid, Dr. Hlawacek gives minute instructions as to how they should act in matters of lesser moment. He is so considerate as to explain how they ought to dress themselves. Their clothing, according to him, should be neither too heavy and warm, nor too tight and light, the compression of the body being injurious, a piece of information which most persons may have acquired before going to Carlsbad and reading the book which Dr. Hlawacek wrote for the benefit of those who are patients there. Even in the summer months one cannot count upon settled weather at Carlsbad. The morning may be warm and still; the afternoon may be cold and stormy. Rain may fall when it is least expected. Hence Dr. Hlawacek advises the patients to bring warm clothing with them, or to provide themselves with it after their arrival. At Carlsbad, as elsewhere, it is prudent to carry an umbrella. There is a Spanish saying to the effect: " Carry an umbrella when it is fine; when it rains do as you please." It is not necessary to know Spanish or to have read Dr. Hlawacek's book to understand that an umbrella is a protection if not a sort of insurance against rain.

Young people, and many who are no longer young, like to be amused at a watering-place. For their gratification a ball takes place weekly in the Curhaus during the season; the theatre is open nightly. No objection is made by Dr. Hlawacek to theatre-going; but his verdict on dancing is a qualified one. Like eating and drinking, he thinks that dancing should be practised in moderation: King Solomon never uttered wiser words. Possibly King Solomon would have agreed with the conclusion of Dr. Hlawacek that dancing is not injurious, as a gentle movement of the body acts beneficially. He is in doubt whether smoking may be permitted. He thinks that the patients who have been in the habit of smoking may continue the practice. He did not know, as a colleague did after he had departed this life, how difficult it was to lay down an absolute rule on this head. A patient listened with attention to what his physician at Carlsbad ordered him to do. "One cigar only a day, after dinner," was the command of the doctor, who added a strict injunction against excess in smoking. After a few days' time the patient returned to the doctor to report progress. "Well," said the doctor, "have you strictly adhered to my orders about smoking?" "Yes, doctor," was the reply; "but I have always been sick afterwards." "How so," said the doctor, "surely you cannot have confined yourself to a single cigar; for if you did, you would not be sick?" "But, doctor, I never smoked before; and, if you do not object, I should prefer to give up the cigar after dinner, as it always makes me sick."

In these days, as in those when Dr. Hlawacek practised, his rules with regard to the rooms in which patients live have lost none of their applicability. He advised patients to live in rooms which are light, airy, and free from draughts and damp. He also objected to patients taking medicine whilst at Carlsbad. The mineral water ought to suffice for all reasonable purposes in the cases of persons whose business is to taste and test it.

I.

Goethe has finely said that a place is consecrated where the immortals have dwelt. This is true of Carlsbad, and he is the immortal. Many days of Goethe's life were spent in Carlsbad and some of his best works were written there. When he visited it in 1785, for the first time, he was thirty-six years old: he was seventy-four when, in 1823, he saw it for the last time. The readers of G. H. Lewes's life of the great poet will not learn anything of his indebtedness to Carlsbad and his love for it. A chapter on that subject would have rendered the work of Lewes still more admirable. The first to give due attention to this matter was the Dr. Hlawacek whose book on Carlsbad has already been referred to and quoted. He composed a small work, entitled, "Goethe in Carlsbad," which appeared in 1877; a second and enlarged edition appeared in 1883, under the editorship of Dr. Victor Nuss. I shall extract the salient and more interesting facts from the second edition.

Goethe suffered in early life from an internal malady, and it was with a view to obtain relief that, for the first time, he journeyed to Carlsbad in 1785; afterwards he visited it many times at intervals for the sake of his health. Writing to Frau Von Stein after his arrival in 1785, he said that the waters which he drank and in which he bathed suited him very well, that being thrown into close contact with his fellows exercised a good effect on him, having helped to "rub off the rust" which had accumulated owing to his life of seclusion, and that all things had contributed, particularly the ladies, to render his stay interesting and beneficial.

Returning the following year, he then occupied himself with preparing an edition of his works for the press. His friend Riemer wrote that Carlsbad had made a new man of him. Goethe informed the Duke of Saxe-Weimar that his health had been greatly improved by taking the waters. On the third of September, 1786, he left Carlsbad in good health and spirits to pay his long contemplated visit to Italy. He wrote that he stole away very early in the morning, and without bidding his friends good-bye, in order that they might not tempt him to prolong his sojourn. He did not return for nine years.

In a letter to Schiller, wherein he described his visit in 1795, Goethe wrote that he was welcomed as a distinguished author, but that some persons confounded him with another living writer. A charming lady, he said, told him that she had read his last work with much pleasure, and that *Ardinghello* had highly interested her, that work being a romance by Heinse. In another letter he noted that the waters were effecting a cure, and that he had scrupulously observed the doctor's orders, getting up at five in the morning, passing his days in idleness, going into society and experiencing some adventures. Yet he could not have been wholly idle, as he had written the fifth book of *Wilhelm Meister* and was about to finish the sixth. Eleven years elapsed before Goethe returned to Carlsbad: it was in 1806 that he visited it for the fourth time. He lodged at the "Three Moors," a house to which he afterwards returned, partly, it is alleged, out of a special liking for the landlady, Frau Heillinggötter. The house still remains as it was in those days. Goethe was then fifty-seven. He doubted whether the waters would benefit him, and his visit was entirely due to the advice of his physician. The improvement in his health was so great and speedy that he regretted to have hesitated so long before starting for Carlsbad.

During all these visits Goethe gave much of his

attention to studying the geology of the valley through which the Tepel flows, and wherein Carlsbad stands. He speculated as to the origin of the mineral springs, and he wrote an essay on the "Bohemian Mountain Range," which long served as a guide to explorers. On the 12th of July, 1806, he sent a letter to Herr Voigt, saying: "The waters suit me very well, and if my present state of health would only last, I should not desire to be better. Müller, the lapidary, who is the same old man, has been induced by the new mineralogists to strive after something novel; he has made some very pretty collections, and I shall bring away a set for my cabinet. Up to the present time the visitors' list shows that 542 persons have arrived; as in former years, they belong to all nations, conditions, and creeds, and they all look to the warm springs for the recovery of their health. This year the 'Neubrunn' is the most fashionable spring, being well adapted for the gentler sex." A few days later he informed Frau Von Stein that he was in capital condition, adding: "My health has been re-established without the aid of physic, and solely by drinking and bathing in the waters here." He notes that the number of visitors had increased to 650. He left Carlsbad early in August. All Bohemia was tranquil then. The prevailing quietude caused Goethe to liken it to the Land of

Goshen. Yet the year 1806 was not one of repose for Austria.

Goethe returned to Carlsbad in the year 1807, and then he wrote a pamphlet on the mineralogy of the district, which was printed there. During this visit, he expressed his desire to do whatever lay in his power to benefit a place which had a marked character of its own, and which he liked the more on that account. It had then what some visitors would now consider a drawback, and what others might pronounce an attraction. This was the opportunity for losing money at public gaming tables. There is no opportunity of the same kind to be found now; yet, whilst public gaming is prohibited throughout Austria, the Government lotteries flourish, and yield a profit of twenty million florins. It may be doubted whether public gaming tables cause more widespread demoralisation than public lotteries.

The treatment which Goethe followed in 1807 differed from that of previous years, inasmuch as he gave up drinking the hot water of the Sprudel, and drank the water of cooler springs. During this visit he wrote some of his minor works. His son and the Dukes of Coburg and Saxe Weimar were amongst the visitors.

In 1808 he paid his sixth visit, arriving at Carlsbad on the 15th of May, and leaving on the

15th of September. He went to Franzensbad and spent twelve days there; after finishing the course of treatment, he returned to Carlsbad, where he devoted the remainder of his stay to geological investigations, to sketching and painting, and writing some of his minor works. Goethe says that he worked as hard then as if he had to make his way in the world. A passage in a letter to Knebel shows that he was not a constant reader of the newspapers, his reason for neglecting them being that they contained so much that was false and misleading. Besides, his friends kept him informed about the events of the day. Yet, if he did not read the newspapers immediately after publication, he did not object read them when they were out of date. He brought with him the *Allgemeine Zeitung* for the years 1806 and 1807, and he seems to have taken pleasure in perusing these old newspapers. As a sign of the unsettled times, he notes that strangers were reluctant to talk politics with each other. From a letter to Frau Von Stein we learn that the only industry which is still prosecuted at Carlsbad, that of pin-making, flourished early in the century. In this letter, which is dated the 16th of May, the day after his arrival, Goethe says: "We have arrived here safely, the weather being fine and the roads bad. Spring is just beginning here. Things look as they did three weeks ago in Weimar. I am very well. Along with this I forward a pound of pins. The price is two thalers twelve groschen in coin. Brass wire is so dear. There is such a demand for brass to make cannon that it is not drawn into wire."

Three months later he wrote: "I am well, and I have no reason to be dissatisfied with this summer. I have experienced all conditions of social intercourse, from entire solitude to the greatest noise and bustle and then solitude again. Thus the summer season at a watering-place closely resembles the life of man. It has been the same as regards the weather. The loveliest May days, rain, heat, and damp, misty evenings, giving a foretaste of those of autumn, and the most beautiful moonlight nights succeeding each other; these are to be found everywhere, yet, in the mountain range and valleys of this district, they impress us the more because they affect us in a more characteristic fashion. Sometimes the heat is like that of an oven, and the rain is like a deluge." Amongst the visitors in 1808, the Duke of Gotha attracted attention by his eccentric behaviour. His custom was to make one of his guests the butt of his ridicule and wit; he spared Goethe, who expressed his surprise at the occasional flashes of clever observation and repartee which the duke displayed.

Returning to Carlsbad in 1810, Goethe was present

when the Empress Maria Ludovica arrived, and he wrote verses in her honour which his least discriminating and capable critics praise the most highly. He was greatly vexed to think that he had not been there the year before, when, in the month of September, there was an explosion at the Sprudel, and when two springs, the Schlossbrunn and the Theresienbrunn, ceased to flow for a time. He was not improved in health by this visit. He went to Teplitz, where the baths did him good. He laid the blame upon the bad weather at Carlsbad, and he expressed his regret at having had to leave "a place which he loved so well."

Goethe arrived at Carlsbad for the eighth time on the 17th of May, 1811; he left it on the 29th of June. This was an unusually short stay. His wife followed him, and did not please his admirers there; the ladies, in particular, spoke contemptuously about "Goethe's corpulent better-half." His friend Riemer notes that the rainy days were so many in number as to mar the pleasure of the sojourn. It is still a drawback at Carlsbad that wet days are frequent in the summer.

Very early in May, 1812, Goethe visited Carlsbad for the ninth time; he was the third arrival that season. Shortly after reaching the place where he expected to regain health, he was confined to bed with a severe attack of what he styled his "old complaint," which is now supposed to be an affection of the kidneys. He went to Teplitz for a short time at the request of the Duke of Weimar, returning to Carlsbad, which he did not leave till the 12th of September. During his stay he wrote a part of his *Wahrheit und Dichtung*, a work which he himself termed a "biographical joke." Then it was that he made the acquaintance of William Von Humboldt, who afterwards wrote a letter expressing the great pleasure he had in conversing with him, and intimating how much struck he was with some views concerning Shakespeare which he requested Goethe to commit to writing.

After an interval of five years, Goethe returned in 1818 to Carlsbad. He there made Prince Blücher's acquaintance, and heard Madame Catalani sing. He returned the following year on the 28th of August, that being his seventieth birthday. During this visit Prince Metternich, Count Bernstorff, and Count Kaunitz assembled together to lay the foundation of that Holy Alliance which was the final and desperate effort of the absolute monarchs of Europe to impede the march of freedom.

The Duke of Mecklenburg then provided a pleasant surprise for Goethe, by getting the clock which hung in the house where he was born in Frankfort, and having it hung in the house wherein he lodged at Carlsbad. When Goethe awoke early in the morning, and heard this clock strike the hour, he called to his servant, saying, "A clock has struck which arouses all the memories of my childhood. Is it a dream or a reality?" After rising and learning the truth, he was moved to tears.

The last time that Goethe visited Carlsbad as a patient was in 1820. He was then most active, notwithstanding his advanced age, in researches of all kinds. During the journey he occupied himself in observing and noting in his diary the cloud formations and the particular conditions under which they were produced. He was present at a wedding, the bride and bridegroom being ordinary people, and belonging to the poorer class. He admits that, by conversing with these persons, he obtained a better notion of the real state of Carlsbad than he had done before, having been accustomed, till then, to regard it as a large hospital and hotel. A flying visit was paid to it in 1823, the chief attraction then being Fräulein Ulricke Levetzow, a young and charming lady, who had smitten the poet's too susceptible heart, and who, notwithstanding, or perhaps owing to his being seventy-four, received an offer of his hand which she declined. This lady remained single from choice. Sixty years later Fräulein Von Levetzow showed that her remembrance of Goethe had not lapsed after the passing of sixty years. In 1883 a marble bust of Goethe, the first erected to his honour in Austria, was unveiled at Carlsbad, and then a wreath of camellias, sent by this venerable lady, was placed at its base.

There have been many changes in Carlsbad since Goethe last saw it. If he revisited it, he would not recognise the places where he used to feel at home. Very few of the houses remain as they were in his time, the one called "The Three Moors," in which he stayed more than once, being an exception; yet others built near to it interfere with the view and render the house a less desirable place of abode. All the houses wherein he lodged, or those which now stand on their sites, have inscriptions setting forth a fact of which their owners are proud. Another man of note in his day, but whose services to mankind are not comparable to Goethe's, is amongst those of whom the sojourn in Carlsbad is commemorated in the like manner. This is the Czar Peter, who is commonly called Peter the Great.

The particulars relating to the visits of the Czar Peter were collected by the chief priest Kustodieff, and narrated to a meeting of Russians held in Carlsbad to commemorate the Czar's two hundredth birthday. His first visit was paid in 1711, when he drank the waters to cure some ailment of which no record is preserved. A picture is extant which shows the manner in which the illustrious patient underwent the treatment. He is represented in bed, and a board is hanging against the wall of the room, on which there are three rows of figures. In the second row the figures 23 are legible. A story is current which may explain the reason for using this board to keep a note of the number of glasses drank. When the doctor first saw the Czar he prescribed three glasses of the water by way of a beginning. The Czar understood him to mean three pitchers, and he selected out of the pitchers used for bringing water from the Sprudel to the house in which he lodged, those which were to be filled for him. He had swallowed the contents of one pitcher, and was beginning to empty a second, when the doctor entered. The Czar said to him: "I think I can manage a second pitcherful, but I cannot possibly get down a third." The doctor was astounded, and hastened to stop this frightful excess in drinking. As the archives of Carlsbad were destroyed by fire in 1759, many of the particulars of the Czar's sojourn are lost. It is known, however, that he was as assiduous at his devotions as in drinking mineral water. There being no Greek Church there in those days, the Czar was in the habit of ascending daily the mountain side, and saying his prayers before a cross, whilst his attendants kept intruders away.

The Czar had a taste for building houses as well as ships. Once he worked as a common mason at Carlsbad, and once he competed for a prize as a marksman. Whilst amusing himself by helping to build a house he took offence, owing to the manner in which a workman regarded him. Being both quick-tempered and free, as he thought, to do what he pleased, he threw a trowelful of mortar in the poor man's face. The man was blinded. The fiery Czar learned afterwards that the man had no intention of seeming to be disrespectful, but that he was astonished to see so great a man as the Czar condescend to work like a common mason. The explanation satisfied and flattered the Czar, and he made the man a present by way of compensating him for the mistake.

This powerful and sensitive ruler had another experience of a like kind in Carlsbad. Going to a place where several marksmen were trying to excel each other in shooting at a target, he joined them, and did his best to gain the victory. A spectator was so much impressed with the Czar's good shooting that he applauded loudly. The Czar, thinking the noise was intended to make him miss, turned his gun upon the enthusiastic spectator and fired at him.

Happily, the shot did not take effect. When informed of his mistake, he made amends by a gift. Apparently, it was nearly as dangerous to applaud the Czar Peter as to oppose any of his whims.

An annual prize of twelve florins and twenty-five kreutzers in money is still competed for by the sharpshooters at Carlsbad. The origin of the prize, as the chief priest Kustodieff remarks, is very curious. It was the result of a gift being wrongly addressed. When the Czar Peter was at Carlsbad the Emperor Charles the Sixth sent him a present of 960 bottles of good Rhine wine. The case containing the bottles was labelled to "His Majesty the Czar Peter." He took offence at this, having intimated that he desired to be addressed as Emperor. He returned the gift. Shortly afterwards the Bohemian Legislature sent him a present of wine, which he handed over to the riflemen as a prize to be shot for. The Czar competed for the prize and won it. He presented the wine to the governing body, with the request that it should be set apart as an object for competition. The wine was sold, and the money thereby obtained yields the interest which is now competed for on the Czar's birthday.

A few mementoes of the Czar's stay at Carlsbad are in good preservation and are less open to objection than some stories of what he did in his haste. Amongst them are an ivory snuff-box and the legs of a table fashioned with his hands at a turning lathe. A spot on the hill slope to the left of the valley, up which he rode on a bare-backed horse, is named after him. Most noteworthy, however, of the circumstances connected with the Czar Peter's visits to Carlsbad was that, when he returned in 1712 for the second time, he then renewed and continued his acquaintance with Leibnitz, which he had begun in 1711 at Torgau. He took counsel at Carlsbad with the great philosopher as to the reforms to be made in Russia. He elevated Leibnitz to the dignity of a privy counsellor, with a yearly salary of 1000 thalers, or £150. Leibnitz gave the Czar much good advice in return; but not even a philosopher like Leibnitz, nor a well-meaning Czar like Peter, can transform a people by a formula or a ukase. Hence it is, that the habits and manners of the Russian people have remained almost unaffected by the understanding arrived at between the philosopher who could frame plausible theories and the Czar who was incapable of patiently applying them in practice.

II.

Many visitors to Carlsbad have left behind them tokens of their gratitude for the benefit received. Instead of writing their names on wooden benches, carving them on trees, or cutting them in stones, they have employed artists to paint their names and their effusions in prose or verse on metal plates, which are affixed to rocks or trees. A granite obelisk, erected in 1883, bears inscriptions in Hungarian, French, and German, to the effect that it is a thank-offering to Carlsbad from grateful Hungarians. In 1859, Kiss, the noted Prussian sculptor, carved an image in the solid rock as a testimony of his skill and good wishes.

Count Findlater has a leading place amongst those persons who have left permanent memorials of their love for Carlsbad. A monument in stone marks the esteem in which the burghers hold his memory. At the end of the last century he devoted much money to improving the walks through the wood which covers the left side of the valley. Moreover, he erected there in 1801 a covered resting-place for weary wayfarers, wherein he placed an inscription in French, expressing his gratitude for living under "the mild and paternal laws of Austria." A gift from an Englishwoman, the Lady Henrietta Maria Stanley of Alderley, deserves mention. It consists of two stone seats at the roadside in front of the English Church. The dates 1842, 1878, are cut in the back of one seat as well as the following lines :

> To the bright town that gave me health and rest
>   Year after year in life's quick pilgrimage,
> Grateful I dedicate these seats, a nest
>   Where youthful love may talk, and wayworn age,
> Remembering all that life has lost and given,
> May pause and think upon the rest of heaven.

In the back of the other seat are chiselled a few beautiful lines by Goethe, expressing in exquisite words how, for all toilers, there is rest at last.

Amongst the walks through the wood on this mountain slope there is one bearing the name of Russell. It was made at the expense of two nephews of the late Earl Russell, who lived at Carlsbad with their mother in early life. One was Arthur, the other Odo Russell. The latter became Lord Ampthill before his sudden and lamented death as British Ambassador at Berlin. He was on the point of starting for Carlsbad before his decease. Previous visits, during which he drank the waters, had proved of great benefit to his health, and it is possible that, if he had been spared to pay another, his life might have been prolonged.

The picturesque walks in all directions form the chief attractions of the place. Most patients are ordered to take "plenty of exercise." Indeed, walking in the open air is a part of the cure. Many of them are too stout for their comfort, and they look forward with satisfaction to a diminution in their weight. Weighing machines abound, and a frequented walk along the river side is lined with them. When a man or woman cannot earn a livelihood in any other way, he or she gets a weighing machine and touts for custom.

Along the roads and in the woods the abundance of small birds strikes those who know how scarce birds are in other parts of the Continent. The Carlsbaders are so fond of birds that a society exists for providing them with food in the inclement wintry weather when food is scarce. The killing of the birds is expressly forbidden. In consequence of this the birds are very tame. Like little boys, small birds are always hungry. Any one sitting down and distributing a few crumbs is soon surrounded with birds eager to be fed.

In Dr. Burney Yeo's work on "Climate and Health Resorts," it is said of Carlsbad: "As the Jewish race tends fatally to obesity, and as the Carlsbad waters possess the property of making fat people thinner, there are always great crowds of fat Israelites here from Germany, Hungary, and Poland." It is perfectly true that stout people of various nationalities

FREQUENTERS OF THE SPRINGS.

and races are conspicuous here, but I do not think that the members of the Jewish race attract special notice unless they are numbered amongst the Polish Jews. These Jews are certainly noteworthy and notorious. They dress as Shylock is represented to have done, and if he were as little given, as they seem to be, to using soap and water, he must have been an even more unpleasant personage than Shakespeare has depicted him. They are more assiduous in drinking the water than bathing in it. They can be smelt as well as seen. Though the outrages of which they are the victims in parts of the European Continent, at the hands of ignorant and jealous peasants and of persons who cannot plead ignorance in extenuation of their bigotry and brutality, render these poor Jews objects of sympathy, yet it is probable that their persistence in dressing as well as acting differently from other people contributes to make them the targets for scorn and attack.

There are many Austrian and a few German officers and soldiers amongst the frequenters of the Carlsbad springs. The presence of Austrian soldiers and officers is largely due to a military hospital having been established here. It is a large and commodious structure. An inscription on the outer wall tells those who pause to read it, that the hospital is dedicated to the Austrian army by a grateful country. Begun on the 18th of August, 1855, it was opened on the 31st of June, 1865. Dr. Gallus Ritter von Hochberger, a Carlsbad physician, who is still hale after reaching his eighty-sixth year, was the prime mover in establishing this hospital and obtaining subscriptions. Money was freely subscribed, not in Carlsbad only, but in other parts of the Austro-Hungarian Empire. The hospital is a large and fine building. Not only are there baths in it, but there is a mineral spring within its precincts.

III.

Though the season proper begins in May and closes at the end of October, there are patients at Carlsbad all the year round. Those who suffer from diabetes, for which the water is the nearest approach to a cure which has yet been discovered, go to Carlsbad at all seasons of the year in the hope to obtain an alleviation of their malady. Yet the number of patients in winter is small, not exceeding fifty at a time. The climate being severe, no one would pronounce Carlsbad a pleasant health resort in the colder months. Even in the height of summer the weather is changeable and sometimes very trying, extreme heat frequently alternating with extreme cold. As has been said already, a good deal of rain falls during the summer months.

Of late years, 30,000 persons have spent three weeks and upwards in Carlsbad during the season. At the middle of the last century the number of visitors did not exceed 300. When Goethe visited it in 1785 for the first time, the number was under 500. Part of the explanation of the increase lies in the simple fact that there were no railways in those days. Yet before the railway was opened in 1870, the number of visitors had risen to 14,000.

As the facilities for reaching Carlsbad were multiplied, the life there underwent a transformation. The society became less select. Persons of title and persons of royal blood did not cease to frequent it, but they were elbowed by others who had neither an inherited nor an acquired title to notice. Shopkeepers with impaired digestions, or poor Jews with enlarged livers, have as much right to go to Carlsbad for relief as they have to invoke the help of a skilled physician; yet when they flock in crowds to any place it becomes less attractive to the fastidious. Magnates and millionaires, who think that the world has been made for their own gratification, complain that Carlsbad has been spoiled by becoming popular. On the other hand, it is indubitable that the alleviation afforded to human suffering and the many cures wrought increase the attraction of Carlsbad a thousandfold. All sorts and conditions of men and women can now profit by its healing springs.

The visitors are no longer welcomed with the formalities which were practised and paid for when the visit to Carlsbad was difficult and costly. In the olden time the arrival of a visitor was announced by a watchman on the top of the town hall, who blew his horn to celebrate the occurrence and give him a reason for demanding payment for his trouble. A band gave the new-comer a serenade. A similar custom prevailed in England for some time after this century began. When a distinguished personage landed at a seaport the church bells rang merry peals in his honour, and the bell-ringers waited upon him afterwards and gave vent to uncomplimentary phrases if he did not pay them handsomely. The blowing of horns and the playing of bands at Carlsbad was followed by applications for gratuities. This custom ended in 1852. From that time till the present it has been the rule for each visitor to pay a fixed sum, which is devoted to maintaining the springs and the bands of music which play at them every morning. The maximum charge for the course of three weeks is fifteen florins. Medical men and paupers are exempted from this tax.

If the question be put, " Who should visit Carlsbad

as a patient?" the answer must be given by a qualified physician. In these days many physicians of the highest rank in Ireland, Scotland, and England have made a special study of the Carlsbad waters, and are thoroughly well qualified for giving advice to those who seek it. Those only who meditate shortening their days by some act of folly should go to Carlsbad and drink the waters there without medical advice.

Dr. Hufeland, whose "Art of Prolonging Life" used to be a favourite work, wrote in 1815 in strong praise of the Carlsbad waters with regard to diabetes, one of the maladies in which ordinary medicine can effect little. Professor Seegen, a distinguished member of the medical faculty of Vienna, and who, for upwards of a quarter of a century, was the principal physician at Carlsbad during the season, has confirmed Hufeland's views as to the value of these waters in arresting the progress of that malady. Indeed, Carlsbad has been styled a vast hospital for diabetic patients. Gout, rheumatism, neuralgia, and dyspepsia are amongst the many ills for which thousands visit Carlsbad for relief, and of which they are often cured there. I repeat, however, that each individual case depends upon circumstances of which the skilled physician is the best judge.

The principal mineral springs are sixteen in

number, and the resemblance between most of them, as regards their ingredients, is very close. Yet the action of each spring is by no means identical. This is the reason why the advice of a physician on the spot is indispensable. The patient who trusts to the light of Nature may do himself harm by drinking one spring, and may derive marked benefit when ordered to drink another. All the springs in ordinary use are warm. The temperature varies. The action of the water upon the system and upon particular maladies is influenced by the heat of the water. The Sprudel, which is the hottest, has a temperature of 165° Fahrenheit; the Kaiser Carl is comparatively cool, its temperature being 102°. The temperature of many others ranges between that of these two.

The waters of Carlsbad are alkaline, but they are not, as is commonly supposed, violent purgatives, their effect being to regulate the functions of the human economy. It would not enlighten the general reader if a list of the ingredients was given; suffice it to say that sixteen have been discovered. The taste is not unpleasant; when allowed to stand till it has become quite cold, the mineral water does not appreciably differ in taste from common water.

Though the water itself is but slightly purgative, the salt extracted from it is so to a high degree; hence, perhaps, the erroneous conclusion that because Carlsbad salts are powerful in their action, the Carlsbad water must be more powerful still. Whilst the most benefit is derived from drinking the water on the spot and following the régime laid down, yet for those who have done this, much advantage is sometimes gained by drinking the water at home. The quantity exported is very large. A Sprudel soap is also prepared, and it is said to be useful in some skin diseases. Sprudel lozenges, or pastilles, are also in request, resembling those of Vichy in their power to relieve acidity of the stomach.

The accommodation for taking baths is on an extensive scale. What struck Dr. William Ord, when he visited Carlsbad in 1876, must have occurred to others, and that is the absence of a large hotel where persons who had to take a course of baths could do so without leaving the house. A form of bath which is greatly in request now, was not known in the days when Goethe was a sojourner at Carlsbad. This is called a moor bath. It consists of a mineralised peat or moor earth which is found at Soos, the property of Herr Mattoni, near Franzensbad, and of which a supply arrives at Carlsbad every morning by rail. This material is mixed with Sprudel water, the temperature of the mass ranging from 90° to 100° Fahrenheit. The patient remains in this thick and dark compound for twenty minutes, and then enters a bath of ordinary water in order to be cleansed. Though the bath is not inviting in appearance, the sensation caused by it is agreeable. Much comfort is afforded by the use of such a bath in cases of rheumatism and affections of the skin.

There is no lack of lodging-houses and hotels at Carlsbad. The population numbers 12,000, and when the season is at its height the visitors are scarcely less numerous. Nearly every private house is prepared for the accommodation of several visitors. Though there are upwards of twelve hotels, yet most of the regular visitors prefer to lodge in private houses. Restaurants and *cafés* abound, and no one needs complain of the fare or the cooking, though the prices may cause legitimate grumbling. In the Carlsbad restaurants, as in those throughout Austria, a custom prevails of paying a small sum to three attendants, in addition to paying largely for the food and wine. The waiters get no wages, and depend altogether for a livelihood upon the generosity of those whom they serve. What appears absurd is that the one who does nothing, except receive payment for one's dinner or supper, expects the largest gratuity. The waiter who takes the order and serves at table expects a smaller sum, and the boy who brings a bottle of water or wine looks for a still smaller sum. Why three persons should have to be paid by those who enter a Carlsbad restaurant is a problem which I have not yet been able to solve.

Ample provision is made for the religious wants of the visitors. In addition to the Roman Catholic church which most of the Carlsbaders frequent, there is a synagogue, a Russian church, and two Protestant churches. The amusements are simple, consisting chiefly of concerts at different hours of the day. In the evening the theatre is open, and it is a building which does credit to the place. The most interesting sight during the season is to be witnessed on the eve and on the day of the Emperor's birthday, the 18th of August. On the night of the 17th the town and the surrounding heights are illuminated. On the day itself there is a parade of the Carlsbad volunteers, which is followed by a service in the church, at the close of which Haydn's magnificent hymn to the Emperor is sung; and in the afternoon there is a banquet in the Curhaus, at which the Burgomaster presides, and at which any visitor who chooses to pay for a ticket may be present. The speech-making after the banquet is not wearisome, being confined to the toast of the Emperor's health. I must state as the result of my experience, that I never heard a toast of the kind given better and more concisely than by Herr Eduard Knoll, the present Burgomaster, nor could it have been received in any gathering with greater enthusiasm.

I have said that all those who go to Carlsbad for treatment should consult a doctor. The only difficulty that may be experienced is whom to consult, seeing that the names of fifty-nine physicians and surgeons are to be found on the official list of those who practise during the season. As the physicians in the largest practice understand English, visitors from England and America have no difficulty in explaining their symptoms. The proportion of English-speaking visitors is small. Out of the 30,000 who were patients at Carlsbad last season, not more than 2,000 had their homes in the United Kingdom, the United States, Canada, or Australia.

Dr. Macpherson, in his "Baths and Wells of Europe," styles Carlsbad the most striking of all the baths. In some respects it is unique. Those who cannot regain their health elsewhere, often return from it cured. Yet some visitors who arrive with great expectations leave it with heavy hearts. In 1611, Rudenius wrote that the waters of Carlsbad will not cure illnesses which are due to magic and witchcraft; this being equivalent to affirming that they will not work miracles. What was true in 1611 is equally true now. It is also true that the good effect is seldom felt at the time, so those who are not appreciably benefited whilst drinking and bathing in Carlsbad water should still retain their faith in the treatment. Their time and substance may not have been wasted in a vain quest after health. They can console themselves with the expectation, which the Carlsbad physicians encourage, that the real good is to be gained and felt after many days. Thus the patients who exult in the plenitude of restored health, and those who anticipate a like blessing in the future, may depart with hearts nearly as light as their purses, after having undergone a "cure" at Carlsbad, the beautiful and beneficent Queen of Bohemian Watering-places.

CHAPTER II.

GIESSHÜBL-PUCHSTEIN.

Seven miles and a half to the north-east of Carlsbad, in a beautiful valley of the river Eger, is the small watering-place of Giesshübl-Puchstein. It is one of the places visited by all the sojourners at Carlsbad. An omnibus runs to it twice daily during the season. The scenery along the road which skirts the Eger for a part of the way is very picturesque. The ground is undulating, and this has prevented a tramway being constructed between the two places. The river is too full of rocks and rapids to allow of a steam-vessel passing along it, and the cost of rendering the river navigable would be very great. Yet by going a short distance out of the direct road it would be possible to connect the two places by rail. Indeed the ground has been surveyed, and it is possible that a railway may be constructed some day. Should this be done many persons would prefer living at Giesshübl-Puchstein to living at Carlsbad, the air in the former place being more bracing, and they might make the short journey in the morning from Giesshübl-Puchstein to drink at the Carlsbad springs. The mineral springs for which Giesshübl-Puchstein is celebrated belong to the category of those table waters which have become so popular in England of late years. But the waters best known and most used in England chiefly come either from France or from some place on or near to the Rhine. Throughout the vast Austro-Hungarian Empire, Italy, Turkey, and Russia, no table water is more in demand than Giesshübler. The visitors to Carlsbad are recommended to drink it at their meals, and the water is so pure and agreeable that those who have drunk it prefer it to any other. It is reputed also to be a most wholesome as well as a very pleasant beverage.

Though the general use of this table water is of comparatively recent date, the existence of the springs from which it is taken has been known for centuries. Dr. Payer and Dr. Summer, two physicians who wrote about Carlsbad as a watering place, the former in 1522, the latter in 1571, both advise patients at Carlsbad to drink Giesshübler also. When the Archduchess Ferdinand took baths at Carlsbad, in 1571 and 1574, she drank this water. Indeed, in the olden days, when it was the custom at Carlsbad to use the mineral water for bathing exclusively, patients seem to have taken Giesshübler as an adjunct to the "cure." Now that patients both bathe in and drink Carlsbad water, they still find benefit from quenching their thirst and diluting their wine with sparkling Giesshübler. It is curious to note how a water so much valued should have been almost forgotten for a time outside of a narrow circle. There has been always a demand for it at or near to the spot, and for nearly a century it has been supplied to the Court at Vienna, yet the quantity exported to a distance was very trifling between the years 1805 and 1829. The reason assigned is the imperfection with which it was then bottled. Since the beginning of this century the art of bottling sparkling mineral waters has been brought to a perfection previously unattainable. In consequence of this, Giesshübler can now be sent to any distance and kept for any time in the same condition as it is when bottled on the spot.

While many physicians and chemists have written about this water from the sixteenth to the nineteenth century, the writer who has been most serviceable in making it appreciated is Dr. Löschner, physician to the Emperor of Austria, who was raised for his services in that capacity to the rank of baron, and who, in 1846, first wrote a paper upon this water. The eleventh edition of Baron Löschner's small work on Giesshübl-

Puchstein is now before me, and from it I extract the following particulars about the rise and progress of the place. Till 1829 not much was done to render Giesshübl-Puchstein attractive. It was then difficult of access, and the few persons who went thither found little to tempt them to remain. Baron Von Neuberg, who became the proprietor of the extensive estate in which the springs are situated, erected a bath-house in 1829, and he arranged for bottling the water in the most improved method. He also made walks through the woods, and his efforts, combined with the writings of various physicians in praise of the water, led to the place being largely visited. Patients went to Giesshübl-Puchstein then, as they do now, not so much to drink the water as to benefit by the climate. Situated about 1500 feet above the sea, the air of the place is very bracing, and it has become celebrated as one wherein what the Germans style an "air cure" can be enjoyed.

In 1852, the principal spring was named King Otto's Spring, after the Sovereign who did not fulfil the expectations which had been formed of him when chosen to be the King of the Hellenes. This spring flows from a cleft in the granite rock forming the slope of the valley on the right side of the river Eger. The point at which the water issues is 110 feet above the river. It is bottled on the spot, and no addition is made in the shape of carbonic acid gas. In this respect Giesshübler has an advantage over the many table waters to which that gas is added artificially. Nature has made it rich enough in carbonic acid gas to be sparkling and pleasant to the palate, and any water in its purely natural state is vastly superior to one which is charged with that gas by artificial means. Indeed, Giesshübler has all the characteristics, without any of the drawbacks, of a natural soda-water. Not till 1873, when the property passed into the hands of Herr Mattoni, of Carlsbad, did the water of Giesshübl-Puchstein begin to be generally appreciated, and to be in large demand outside the limits of Bohemia.

Herr Mattoni, who holds the rank of Imperial Councillor, belongs to a family of Italian origin which settled in Carlsbad. Having determined both to develop the resources of Giesshübl-Puchstein and to beautify it, Herr Mattoni improved the roads and made walks in the neighbourhood, built villas for the accommodation of visitors, and erected baths of the most modern kind for carrying out the hydropathic system of treatment. The result has been that many persons resort to Giesshübl-Puchstein for treatment during the season, while the visitors to it who spend a day there number about 20,000. A physician from Prague, who regularly spends the season there, gives medical advice to the patients. There is good fishing in the Eger and smaller streams flowing into it, the principal fish in the river being carp and pike, whilst trout abound in its tributaries. In the autumn, partridges, hares, and larger game are abundant.

For beauty of situation, Giesshübl-Puchstein is surpassed by few places. In quietness it occupies an equally high place; yet those persons who go to a watering-place for amusement may think it far too quiet. A band plays twice a week; concerts and theatrical performances take place at intervals; the other amusements are walking in the woods, and rowing on or fishing in the river. Its charms, then, are chiefly supplied by Nature. These are sufficient for many persons who return here season after season. Indeed, this small place possesses all the natural attractions of Carlsbad in bygone days, when the houses were fewer in number, and the buildings less imposing; when the air was purer, owing to the absence of chimneys from which dense smoke ascends; before hundreds of trees had been felled to make room for houses, and before green paths were covered with paving stones.

The business of bottling and preparing the water of Giesshübler for exportation gives employment to upwards of 200 persons. The consumption of wood in the packing-cases is an important item; and in order to provide the wooden boards Herr Mattoni has a sawmill at work during a part of the year. He is most liberal in allowing visitors to visit every part of his large and well-ordered establishment. The processes are many and the mechanical arrangements are as complete as can be desired. The bottles which have been filled and corked at the King Otto's Spring descend in a truck on an inclined railway, one truck ascending while another is descending. In a spacious room at the bottom they are labelled and capsuled and packed in wooden cases. As many as 20,000 can be filled in a day. A noteworthy and ingenious arrangement is that for cleaning the bottles. They are placed singly, neck downwards, on tubes through which a current of water issues under heavy pressure, the current being mixed with fine sand, and in this way every impurity inside each bottle is removed. Each bottle undergoes a second process of the like kind, in which water only is used, and it is then placed in a tank of water. The cleansing machine is the invention of a Carlsbad engineer, and is the most effective one of the kind yet introduced. Having tried many others, Herr Mattoni gives this one the preference.

The demand for Giesshübler increases yearly. At

the beginning of the century not more than 80,000 bottles were exported; the number had increased to 150,000 in 1834. When Herr Mattoni began to improve upon the methods of bottling the water ten years ago, the demand for it did not exceed 300,000 bottles. Five years later the number sold was 3,000,000 yearly, and last year it rose to upwards of 5,000,000. This water tastes exactly like the best spring water. What renders it beneficial to the system is the fact of its containing minute quantities of chemical substances, all of which, in combination, not only taste pleasantly, but tend to promote health. The entire absence of salt from this water is greatly in its favour, the presence of salt in other table waters being an objection to their frequent use. The proportion of the bicarbonates of soda and potass is noteworthy. The quantity of natural carbonic acid gas makes it sparkle. Mixed with wine, spirits, or fruit syrups, Giesshübler forms an agreeable and refreshing drink. Chemists in the first rank, of whom Liebig is one, and physicians of the highest class, amongst whom Dr. Garrod may be named, have written strongly in praise of Giesshübl water. There is the less need to quote what has been said and printed in commendation of it, as the great and increasing demand is conclusive evidence as to its popularity. It is not so well known in England and America as some other table waters. When the public shall have become better acquainted with it in both countries, the demand for Giesshübler will probably become as large as it is throughout the continent of Europe.

Though the spring named after King Otto is the one from which the most water is drawn, yet there are three others which can be brought into use when required. These are named Elizabeth, Francis Joseph, and Löschner. The water from the first has been valued under the name of "Rodisfort" for a long time. It issues from the ground near a small stream which, when in flood, overspreads the surface. As a result of this, as well as of the earth mixing with the water whilst it rose to the top, the spring was not of much use. However, Herr Mattoni caused a boring to be made in the granite, through which the mineral water now rises pure and fitted for bottling. The temperature of this spring is a few degrees higher than the Otto; in consequence of this the carbonic gas escapes more rapidly when a bottle containing the water is opened, and gives the impression of being more highly charged with gas than the others. Yet the constituents of both are almost identical. Though a large quantity of the Elizabeth is bottled to meet the increasing demand, yet it is estimated that as much mineral water runs away into the stream as would fill many millions of bottles.

Francis Joseph, a spring not far from the Elizabeth, is used for the purpose of supplying baths. The Löschner, which is the last that has been discovered here, has not yet been analysed or turned to account.

Enough has been written to show that the place where Giesshübl water is found has many points of interest. It is well worth a visit. Many who go there to spend a day feel disposed to remain for a longer time. That Giesshübl-Puchstein will grow and become still more frequented is most probable. But I cannot help repeating that it will not gain in attractiveness by increasing in size. Now is the time to see it at its best. Amongst the smaller baths of Bohemia, there is not a prettier or more picturesque one than Giesshübl-Puchstein.

CHAPTER III.

FRANZENSBAD.

When a paragraph used to appear in the newspapers that the late Prince Gortchacoff purposed visiting Baden-Baden, had arrived here, or had left it, few if any readers were in doubt as to where the place was situated in which the distinguished Imperial Chancellor loved to sojourn. Baden-Baden is one of the health resorts on the European continent about which everybody may be supposed to know something. Its name is as familiar to an Englishman, a Frenchman, an Italian, a Russian, and an American as to the native of the Grand Duchy of which it forms a part.

A few years ago it was announced in the newspapers that M. de Giers, who, as Minister for Foreign Affairs, succeeded to the most important of Prince Gortchacoff's duties, had visited Franzensbad. Many readers might not have had a clear notion as to the place and the way thither. I neither assume nor assert that in these days of universal examinations any one would voluntarily admit lack of knowledge on any point. Yet those who knew the most about everything, and about Franzensbad in particular, might have wondered why M. de Giers should have chosen that watering-place as a place wherein to pursue a course of treatment. Franzensbad has had a long established and a high reputation among Bohemian health resorts; but its frequenters belong so largely to the fairer sex that Franzensbad is commonly regarded as exclusively a ladies' bath. Of late years, however, it has ceased to be visited by fair patients alone. Several eminent German physicians having decided that women should not monopolise the attractions of Franzensbad, they are now in the habit of sending men thither to drink and bathe in its mineral waters. Hence it is that M. de Giers, among others, resorted to that place in order to regain the health which he had lost through protracted overwork in conducting the foreign affairs of the vast Russian Empire.

Franzensbad lies at the north-western extremity of Bohemia. A few miles' journeying in one direction brings one to the frontier of Saxony, and, in another, to the frontier of Bavaria. About five miles distant is the city of Eger, which is situated on the river of the same name. The town of Franzensbad is built upon a slight slope facing southwards. In olden days its site was a barren, marshy, and desolate moor. It may be styled an inland Venice. The ground was so unstable at the surface that no houses could be erected till piles had been driven far down to form a foundation for them; yet the resemblance between Franzensbad and Venice begins and ends at these piles. The surface is covered with sufficient soil to afford an extensive bed for shrubs and trees. Indeed, the houses are scattered about over a vast area, which is covered with plants and flowers, and chestnut and other trees, the foliage being so dense in spring and summer that the houses are hidden behind a screen of leafy branches. The houses are of modern date, and they are comfortably arranged. Though the streets are lit with old-fashioned oil lamps, the houses contain many modern improvements, including electric bells. There are not many more than 150 private houses and hotels, all of them being arranged for the reception of visitors, the rooms available for the purpose being 3000. As many as from 8000 to 9000 persons visit Franzensbad in the season for the purpose of undergoing treatment there.

Though the fame of Franzensbad as a watering-place did not attract many visitors from a distance till the beginning of the present century, yet its mineral waters were in repute, within a limited circle, for a long time previously. A printed reference to one of its mineral springs dates as far back as 1502. The Queen of Poland drank the Franzensbad water in 1629 with a view to benefit her health. But at that time the water was brought to Eger and drunk there. It was not till 1660 that the authorities of the city of Eger allowed an inn to be built at the spring, and not till 1707 was any arrangement made for taking mineral water baths at the place which now bears the name of Franzensbad. The demand for such accommodation grew the more pressing as an increasing number of persons went from Eger to drink the waters.

Dr. Bernard Adler, who was impressed with the medicinal value of these mineral waters, determined to render the place whence they issued from the ground more comfortable for drinking purposes, and, with that view, he caused a suitable structure to be raised over it. The women of Eger were angrily opposed to this innovation; they wished to bring the water to Eger for sale, and they disapproved of people going to drink it in comfort at the spring. On August 18, 1791, a band of these women marched from Eger, and destroyed the building erected by Dr. Adler. Returning in triumph to Eger, they passed the night in singing, dancing, and drinking beer.

Had not Dr. Adler concealed himself, the infuriated women might have taken his life. When the ringleaders were apprehended, the others crowded before the magistrate and exclaimed that they were all parties to the act of destruction, the result being that they were all suffered to go free. However, Dr. Adler persevered in his design, and he succeeded a few weeks later in getting the consent of the Emperor to the spot being officially recognised as a wateringplace. Permission was not only given by the Emperor to the effect that people might settle and build houses, but special privileges were also conferred upon the first settlers on the site of Franzensbad. The final arrangements were made in 1793, when a plan of the town was drawn up, and this plan was carefully followed till the year 1849. In 1793, the place was formally named Franzensbad, after Francis the First, then Emperor of Austria.

Whilst the spring first discovered at Carlsbad, which is known as the Sprudel, still continues to be the most important, at Franzensbad the first spring which attracted attention is now regarded as of less value than some of the others. In 1808 the Louisenquelle was discovered and turned to account. Close to it the Cold Sprudel, as it is called, was found in 1818. A year later the Salzquelle, a spring which is now highly valued, was first used, and its virtues were so marked that, within seven years after its discovery, as many as 30,000 bottles of it were exported annually. The water of the Wiesenquelle was very little appreciated till 1837. Most noteworthy as an iron spring is the Stahlquelle, which was not discovered till 1860. This spring is even stronger in iron than those of Schwalbach and Spa. It is clear, then, that out of the twelve mineral springs now in use at Franzensbad, many of them have but a brief history, though the place itself was noted for its mineral water three centuries ago.

Bathing is here regarded as an almost indispensable adjunct to water-drinking, and the variety of baths is nearly as great as that of the mineral springs. The four largest bathing establishments, which contain altogether about 450 separate bath-rooms, are called respectively Dr. Loimann's Bath-house, the City of Eger Bath-house, the Cartellieri Bath-house, and the Imperial Bath-house. Till the year 1827, the baths were in private houses. Dr. Loimann built the first public bath-house in that year, adding a second in 1841, which has been greatly enlarged since then. The Commune of Eger built one in 1850; Dr. Cartellieri built one in 1863, which he enlarged in 1869; whilst the Imperial Bath-house, which is a handsome edifice externally, was constructed within the last few years.

There are three different kinds of baths in general use: the mineral water baths, the gas baths, and the moor baths.

A few years ago, when the patients were chiefly ladies, the arrival of a gentleman at Franzensbad excited general attention. The newcomer was in as enviable a position as David Hume during his sojourn in Paris as secretary to the British Embassy. All the Parisian beauties were at his feet; no fine lady thought an entertainment complete unless he were present. He was asked to play the part of a sultan, but he miserably failed to do justice to it. What made him the rage was his reputation as an historian and a philosopher, and in the year 1763, all the beautiful and accomplished ladies of Paris were ardent admirers, if not readers, of history and philosophy. At Franzensbad, however, a gentleman used to be in request, not solely on account of his merits, but his rarity. He was a sort of black swan or white crow. The proportion of male to female patients was then as one in a hundred. Now that there are five men out of every hundred patients, the attention paid to gentlemen by ladies has sensibly diminished.

Many of the ladies are young, and all of them seem delicate. What strikes one as unusual is the independent manner in which they conduct themselves. At home they would probably object to go alone into a restaurant or *café*, and order dinner or refreshment, while at Franzensbad every restaurant and *café* is chiefly frequented by ladies, who appear to be quite at their ease. Franzensbad is the watering-place most closely resembling the "Adamless Eden" which has been represented on the stage.

As ladies have greater faith in a doctor than gentlemen, and as they are quite ready to give implicit obedience to a doctor's injunctions, the physicians at Franzensbad find little difficulty in getting their orders obeyed. For this reason, perhaps, they are rather despotic, and the regulations which they enforce are of a minute and elaborate kind. The following is a summary of the rules for passing the day in accordance with medical advice: The patient gets out of bed between five and six in the morning, and reaches the springs not later than six, spending the time between six and eight in drinking water and walking about. Between eight and nine is the time for breakfast. A bath is taken between nine and twelve, and the patient is allowed to read or write letters in the unemployed intervals. The hour for dinner is between twelve and two. An option is given of either making excursions in the neighbourhood on foot and in a carriage between half-past three and eight, or sitting in the open air from half-past three till six, the tedium being relieved either by a cup of coffee at four, or by a glass of mineral water between five and six. Supper is eaten between seven and eight, and the patient goes to bed at nine.

The residents at Franzensbad are made to understand that they must carefully consider and provide for the requirements of the patients there. Lest they should forget this, the authorities have issued an order, of which the following is a literal translation:

No patient must be disturbed at night. To insure quiet, each proprietor of a house must prevent noises occurring, either in the house itself or in the street, between nine at night and six in the morning; on the other hand, the patients are requested, for the sake of others in the houses they occupy, to stop all noisy amusements, such as music, piano-playing, singing, &c., at nine o'clock in the evening.

The physicians at Franzensbad are very particular about the kind and amount of food eaten by patients. Dr. August Sommer strongly warns them against eating too much at a time. What he permits, and others do so likewise, is a very light breakfast of weak coffee, chocolate or cocoa nibs, or boiled milk, with two rusks or small rolls; this being enough, in his opinion, to satisfy the keenest appetite for the moment. Dr. Sommer, Dr. Buberl, and others set their faces against tea-drinking, especially at breakfast, on the ground that tea does not agree with the waters. Though tea is forbidden, notices are conspicuously placed in the restaurants to the effect that tea can be supplied. If the patients are very hungry after having taken a bath, they may relieve their craving for nourishment with a small basin of soup, one or two soft-boiled eggs, or a piece of lean ham, either cooked or raw. For dinner they are allowed a little strong but not rich soup, a piece of trout or pike boiled in salt water, a piece of meat, game, or fowl, a small portion of vegetables, a light pudding or stewed fruit. Between dinner and supper a cup of coffee, chocolate, or a glass of milk may be drunk. At supper the fare may consist of soup, stewed fruit, soft-boiled eggs, or a morsel of fowl or tender steak. Plain water is the beverage recommended at dinner and supper; but, should the weather be very warm, a little soda-water or light beer is permitted, whilst poor-blooded patients may indulge in a little old red wine. Patients who are accustomed to smoke, and they are presumably of the male sex, are told that they may smoke mild cigars in moderation; but they are strictly forbidden to smoke at the springs in the morning, when taking a bath, or immediately before going to bed.

Patients who feel sleepy during the day are warned against taking a nap. They are told that if they go to bed between nine and ten at night and sleep till six in the morning, they have had as much repose as is good for them; the only exceptions being very delicate persons, who, if they get special permission from the doctor, may sleep in a chair for not longer than half an hour during the day. Besides drinking and bathing in mineral water and eating sparingly of very plain food, patients are advised that their cure largely depends upon keeping their minds easy. They are enjoined to preserve an even temper, to dismiss from their thoughts all considerations of business or study, and to beware lest they indulge in excessive grief or joy, or get excited about religion or politics. Lovemaking is discountenanced by the doctors both here and at Carlsbad. They consider that a passion for mineral waters and baths should be absorbing enough to exclude any other of a more ethereal kind. Those who enter Franzensbad are to leave all worries behind them. If this could be done as easily and completely as the physicians suppose, many persons would hasten to Franzensbad.

I readily admit that the temptations to overexcitement at Franzensbad are very few. A band plays twice daily; there is a small theatre, where light pieces are performed between seven and nine in the evening; a ball takes place in the Curhaus every Saturday; and on all days of the week a reading room is open. A German writer about Franzensbad states that the town is as silent as the grave at nine o'clock in the evening, the streets being then deserted, and the visitors being either in or going to bed. My experience is that profound stillness reigns at eight. There is but one large *café* in the town. On the first night of my arrival there, I went to the *café* between seven and eight, to drink a cup of coffee after a light dinner, but I found it closed, business ending at the early hour of seven o'clock. Going to bed early is comparatively easy in Franzensbad, as there is nothing else to do after the simple meal which is there called supper. To rise early is almost a necessity. Whilst silence is maintained during the night, a racket begins at six o'clock in the morning, which effectually banishes sleep.

The noteworthy buildings and monuments in Franzensbad are few in number. There is a Roman Catholic church, a Protestant church, and a Synagogue. A site has been obtained for a Russian church, but the funds for erecting it have not yet been subscribed. In the park there is a bronze statue of the Emperor Francis the First, who encouraged the rise of the new watering-place, and allowed it to be named after him. A monument has also been erected in memory of Dr. Bernard Adler and of Herr Limbeck, the Burgomaster of Eger, both of whom largely contributed to found the town. More useful than any monument, is the hospital for the reception and treatment of forty-five poor patients, without distinction of country or creed, who bring with them a medical certificate that they require treatment, and another as to their poverty. A hospital is established for the reception of poor patients from Mid-Saxony. An asylum for widows and orphans has been erected in memory of Dr. Fürst. There is also an institution for enabling invalid officers in the Austrian army to be treated here, free of charge for living or medical attendance. Many Jews visit Franzensbad, and a fund for the assistance of the poorer ones was established in 1845.

The literature about Franzensbad is rich; I have a list of thirty-four books on the subject. Four of the most noteworthy contain information of present value; they are by physicians in practice here— Dr. Buberl and Dr. Sommer, Dr. Klein and Dr. Cartellieri. These physicians are very emphatic in advising visitors to obtain medical advice and follow it implicitly. Dr. Buberl warns patients who revisit Franzensbad against resuming the course of treatment without consulting a doctor. Whilst it cannot be denied that the systematic way in which the "cure" is conducted at Bohemian watering-places has done much to popularise the Bohemian mineral waters, it should not be forgotten that the waters of the most highly valued places, of which Franzensbad is one, became famous for effecting cures before medical men paid any heed to them. Dr. Sommer is most anxious that all patients should be leisurely in their movements, and should not be impatient to drink so many glasses, bathe so many times, and then rush away. When told by the doctor that they have done their duty as patients, they should wait a few days before starting off, should be in no hurry about packing up, and should not think that they will do themselves any good by taking a farewell glass or bath on the day of their departure. At most of these watering-places the "cure" is supposed to take twenty-one days, but at Franzensbad, according to Dr. Klein, the patients should undergo treatment for six weeks. Some may have stayed the allotted number of weeks, and strictly followed the doctor's orders, yet they may not feel any improvement. For the consolation of such patients Dr. Sommer says that weeks and even months may elapse before the desired benefit is experienced. The visitor to Franzensbad, as well as to other Bohemian watering-places, must exercise patience and self-denial while under treatment, and must live in the hope of better things afterwards.

The situation of Franzensbad is less picturesque

than that of many other Bohemian baths. Though the vast plain, bounded in the far distance by a low range of hills, may appear uninteresting, it has yet a wide reputation for fertility, being known and admired as the rich Egerland. This part of Bohemia is inhabited by 50,000 persons, who are nearly all Teutonic in race, speech, and sentiment. In dialect, customs, and costume, they differ from their neighbours in the German Empire and from the Germans in Austria. They are an industrious people. Farming is their principal occupation, and the farm-houses have a character of their own, being enclosed within walls, as if to protect them from attack. It is the rule for the eldest son to succeed to his father's farm. Though plodding and not very bright, the Egerlanders are fond of amusements, particularly of singing and dancing, and when a wedding takes place the festivities are prolonged for several days. They have many songs and sayings which bear a stamp of originality. A dance called the "Drischlag" is peculiar to this part of the country; it has some resemblance to the polka.

Eger, the ancient Imperial city and fortress, can be reached on foot in an hour and a half; the walk is a very pleasant one, and Eger itself is well worth a visit. Here are the ruins of the old castle built in the reign of the fierce Emperor Barbarossa, within which is a black tower of still earlier date. In the twelfth century, when that castle arose, were laid the foundations of the St. Nicholas's Church, of which the two spires are seen long before Eger itself is visible to pedestrians approaching it from Franzensbad. In Eger the sightseer may visit the house where Wallenstein was murdered by the Irishman Devereux, a tragedy which gave Schiller a theme for the drama which all readers of his works admire, and which Coleridge, by his beautiful version, which is too free to be termed a translation, has rendered familiar to English readers. Yet there are natural phenomena not far distant from Franzensbad which are quite as remarkable as the old city of Eger and its historical associations. One of them, which is on the way thither, is the Kammerbühl, an extinct volcano.

Goethe paid more than one visit to Franzensbad, his first visit being in 1808, as is recorded on a tablet fixed in the wall of the house which he then occupied. He revisited the town in 1811 and 1822. The chief thing which interested him on all these occasions was the Kammerbühl, of which he has left an account. This extinct volcano rises a little more than a hundred feet above the surrounding plain. It is not the view from the top, but the constitution of the elevation itself, which has made it an object of curiosity. There was a time when the surrounding plain was submerged, and when this small volcano may alone have reared its round head above the waste of waters. Appearances indicate that the plain was once the bed of a vast inland lake, and it has been conjectured that the volcano may have become extinct whilst under water. This theory is advanced to explain some appearances which are not easily explicable on any other supposition. The Kammerbühl is supposed to have been active for a short time only.

Many researches have been made, as Dr. Palliardi sets forth in a small but exhaustive work on the subject, to ascertain the inner constitution of this volcano. Shafts have been sunk and levels have been driven towards the interior, but the work was suspended before it had been completed. It would cost a considerable sum to elucidate the mystery of the volcano's constitution, yet the outlay might yield profitable results in the form of scientific facts. The present owner does not appear to care for these things, as he is disposing of the contents of the crater for the purpose of mending roads. In the course of a few years the greater part of the volcano will have disappeared, unless the work of destruction be suspended. As an unique natural curiosity it deserved a better fate.

The prospect from the summit of the volcano chiefly attracts sightseers. There is always a possibility of the interest in it growing more intense and personal. It has been extinct for centuries, but this is no reason against its again becoming active. Vesuvius was pronounced extinct long before the Christian era, and, after an outburst, it remained quiescent between the years 203 and 472. Etna has been silent for four centuries at a time. Should the Kammerbühl again vomit forth flames and smoke, ashes and lava, the visitors to Franzensbad would then experience some novel and not very pleasing sensations, while they would be exposed to an amount of excitement which their physicians might consider highly injurious. It is true that the Kammerbühl is a Liliputian amongst volcanoes, yet even a small volcano, like a small dog, can prove mischievous when in an angry mood.

The other natural phenomenon is at Soos, which is a few miles distant. Here is Herr Mattoni's establishment for extracting the moor earth, wherewith the moor baths at Carlsbad and elsewhere are prepared. The property, which covers an area of several miles, presents an extraordinary appearance. At first sight it would seem to be a piece of barren moorland; but when closely surveyed, the surface is seen to differ from that of any moor. In truth, nothing on the Continent of Europe exactly resembles it except a small tract in Hungary and in the Caucasus. It bears a close likeness on a small scale to some parts of the wonderful Yellowstone region in the United States.

Almost in the middle of Herr Mattoni's property at Soos there is a mineral spring called the Kaiserbrunn, which issues with considerable force from the ground, and this is only one of the many springs which gush forth there. In all directions the ground seems in a ferment with gaseous water. Wherever one stops to listen, bubbling gas is heard issuing from the smallest crack in the soil. All the water is highly mineralised, abounding in glauber salts, iron, and several chemical compounds. The surface is variegated with bright colours, being covered with a white incrustation in some places, and in others having brilliant red and yellow tints. For many feet below the surface the turf is saturated with minerals, and it is this thoroughly mineralised turf which is found to make the best moor baths. Some parts of the ground abound in yellow ochre well fitted for the purification of coal gas, and much of it is exported for the purpose. The mineralised earth, after being dug up, exposed to the air for some time and then dried, is fitted to be used in baths. This earth is treated so to extract the essential elements from it, and the result is so satisfactory that one pound of the concentrated earth serves the purpose of fifty pounds of the cruder kind. The crystallised salts are equally serviceable, and for those who prefer it, a liquid preparation may be obtained. A purgative salt is extracted from the water of the Kaiserbrunn.

I was informed by Herr Roedl, who manages the works here for Herr Mattoni, and who has made a close study of the geology and mineralogy of Franzensbad, that nothing more curious and interesting from a scientific point of view can be found in Bohemia than this moor. It may almost be called a chemical laboratory, in which Nature is producing marvels before one's eyes. In addition to the strange sights which can be witnessed, there are buried treasures of a prehistoric age, quite as remarkable and precious. The bones of extinct animals are found now and then far below the surface, and it is possible that others may yet come to light which will have as great value to the paleontologist as any which have been discovered. One of the latest finds was a large part of the skeleton of a dinotherium, which Herr Mattoni has presented to the Imperial and Royal Museum at Vienna

I ought to state how much I am indebted to Herr Roedl for information most courteously conveyed respecting the processes of rendering the moor earth marketable. He answered all my questions, and allowed me to see everything without hesitation. I learnt from him that the demand for moor lye and moor salt has greatly increased of late years, and that large quantities of both are exported; it having been found that by using either, any one can have all the benefit of a moor bath in his own house. The result has been to enable those persons who do not care, or who cannot make a journey to the places where moor baths are obtainable, to be treated in an hospital or at home.

Few persons visit Franzensbad who do not intend to go through a course of treatment. The number of English visitors is small; indeed, many of the ailments for which the waters of this place are suitable can be treated at Spa or Swalbach. A considerable number of the patients who have drunk and bathed in the powerful waters of Carlsbad come here to enjoy what is called the "after cure." It is a notable peculiarity of Bohemian, as well as of other Continental watering-places, that the "cure" is seldom completed in one of them, and that a second and different course of treatment is required at one place to confirm or compensate for the treatment at another. Certainly, the change from Carlsbad to Franzensbad is not unpleasant. The air at the latter is clear and bracing. Indeed the purity of the air may have nearly as much influence as the waters in restoring tone to the systems of debilitated invalids. A writer on this place quotes statistics to show how healthy it is. He seems proud to record that the death-rate is eighteen in the thousand only. This is low compared with that in many other places on the Continent; but it does not seem so striking to a citizen of the United Kingdom, where the rate in the thousand is but nineteen, and it seems high to a dweller in the London suburb of Kensington, where it is fifteen only. However, the inhabitants of Franzensbad are quite satisfied with their lot, and they have a firm faith that human life is prolonged by the use of the Franzensbad mineral waters. These waters are exported in large quantities. The inhabitants are entitled to refer with satisfaction to a remarkable and most important cure in the case of a mighty monarch. Hufeland records that Frederick the Great got rid of a serious internal malady and preserved his health by drinking the water of the Franzensbrunn.

Not long ago an interesting communication appeared in a Berlin weekly medical journal, from Professor F. T. von Frerichs, one of the leading physicians of the German capital, who had been in the habit of sending patients to Franzensbad during the last thirty-two years. He had not visited the place till he did so as a patient, and he not only derived great benefit from the treatment, but returned home more convinced than ever of the advantages of Franzensbad as a place wherein those who had lost their health might regain it. He wrote with a personal enthusiasm which proves how much he had benefited by his sojourn. It is fair to conclude that he must have been convinced that Franzensbad was a place for men as well as for women who were out of health. When Franzensbad loses the reputation of being almost exclusively a ladies' bath, it will be changed in many respects. I cannot think that women will object to the change; they are too amiable to desire a monopoly of any pleasure or any medicine, and they will not object, I feel confident, to share their enjoyment of Franzensbad with the suffering members of the male sex.

I confess to liking the place far better than I expected. I had read and heard much against it. Its dulness was pronounced intolerable; its situation was styled unattractive. I have seen many livelier and more picturesque watering-places, yet I know of none which appears better adapted for patients who are afflicted with debility, and who require tonic water and bracing air. I have visited it more than once. On the day that I went there for the second time the place was the reverse of dull. The streets were thronged with eager sightseers. The excitement which prevailed betokened that a great event was impending. What occurred was the arrival of Prince Bismarck to confer with Count de Giers, the Russian Minister, as to what should be done in Bulgaria after the revolution which began by Prince Alexander being compelled to depart. The German Chancellor remained three days in Franzensbad; his meeting with the chief Minister of Russia was an historical event of the first importance. Nothing would please the Franzensbaders more than Prince Bismarck's return. They cheered as if they loved him. His visit was a splendid advertisement of the watering-place of which they are proud, and in which the visitors who have plenty of money to spend can find most comfortable lodgings, and restaurants where the food and cooking cannot be surpassed in Austria. If the baths and waters are as efficacious in restoring health as the physicians who know them best represent them to be, then the few drawbacks of the place are so trifling when compared with the final compensation that may well be borne for several weeks without repining.

CHAPTER IV.

MARIENBAD.

When journeying through Bohemia, I was in the compartment of a railway carriage where a fellow-passenger who knew little English was courteously explaining to another, who knew no German, some of the peculiarities and sights of Marienbad. The Englishman seemed perplexed when his travelling acquaintance emphatically told him that Marienbad abounded in "very thick ladies." In reply to a request for an explanation, he only received the further assurance that many ladies were to be seen there who were "so very thick," or, as the last word sounded, so "dick." I cleared up the mystery and misunderstanding by explaining to my fellow-countryman that his German acquaintance wished to tell him that the ladies he would see were very corpulent, and by informing the German that, though he had given a literal translation of the German word, yet that "thick" was never used by the English in the sense intended by him. Though not perfectly clear, the German was perfectly correct in his statement. The sight of so many corpulent ladies is the one which strikes the newcomer at Marienbad. If Hawthorne had visited this place, he would have admitted that Englishwomen are outdone in exceptional rotundity by their Continental sisters. He would have remarked, moreover, that, when an English lady is stout, she is stout symmetrically, whereas many German ladies being excessively stout in parts, seem strangely disproportioned. Besides, an Englishwoman is seldom conspicuous for size till she has reached a mature age, whereas the German and other women who visit Marienbad are still comparatively young, and in this respect the contrast is very marked between their faces and their figures.

Marienbad is one of the four best known and most frequented Bohemian watering-places, and it is the most beautifully situated of them all. Carlsbad has the drawback of being too much shut in; the country around Franzensbad is rather too flat; while Marienbad lies in a very wide valley, encompassed with richly-wooded and finely-shaped hills. At Carlsbad the springs are in the heart of the city, and the paths to be trodden in the intervals of drinking the waters are either under cover or along paved streets. Both at

Franzensbad and Marienbad the springs are in a wood or a garden, and the walks have all the charms which the sight of trees and shrubs, green turf and lovely flowers can impart. Yet these attractions in both places are largely artificial. I described in the last chapter how Franzensbad had been erected on a barren moor, where the soil was so scanty and the ground so moist that piles had to be driven deep down in order to serve as a stable foundation for the houses. The site of Marienbad was a marsh. At present people walk through pleasure gardens where wild beasts formerly roamed.

Though the reputation of Marienbad among watering-places is now very high, yet the virtue of its springs was not generally understood and appreciated till the present century was twenty years old. Its jubilee was celebrated in 1868. That mineral waters existed at Marienbad was known long before they were rated at their present value. Soon after their discovery a great disappointment was caused by their proving to be very different from what was expected. It had been supposed that they were pure saline springs. Common salt was then as greatly prized and costly in Bohemia as it is in Central India now, and a spring yielding salt in abundance was as precious there as the richest gold mine. The Emperor Ferdinand the First, being

AN UNEXPECTED DISCOVERY.

impressed with the great advantage which would accrue to his kingdom of Bohemia if salt were extracted from the Marienbad water, issued a decree on the 27th of April, 1528, ordering a quantity of the water to be bottled and sent to Prague. His commands were obeyed. The water being treated in the usual way when salt is extracted, much salt was obtained; but, to the dismay of those whose expectations had been raised to a high pitch, the salt was found to be that which serves as a purgative medicine, and not that which is employed and esteemed as a condiment. The Marienbad mineral water is very rich in sulphate of soda, or glauber salts. Though this discovery did not gratify the Emperor Ferdinand the First, it had the result of attracting multitudes to Marienbad.

The service which Dr. David Becher rendered to Carlsbad, which Dr. Bernard Adler rendered to Franzensbad, was rendered to Marienbad by Dr. Nehr. He was the physician to Tepel Abbey. The ground on which Marienbad is built and the chief mineral springs there are part of the abbey's domain. Dr. Nehr wrote a description of the place when he first visited it a century ago. No spot could be less attractive. He saw there morasses and heaps of stone, fallen trees and foaming torrents, but no proper arrangement for drinking or bathing in the mineral water. He noted a miserable hut, in which two iron kettles placed over a fire were employed for evaporating the water from the Kreuzbrunnen in order to extract glauber salts, whilst the spring itself, which issued from the ground in the midst of a marsh, was protected by a rude wooden enclosure. Neither footpath nor road led to that spring. It was necessary to leap from stone to stone in the marshy ground to reach it.

Before Dr. Nehr exerted himself in 1779 to improve the arrangements at Marienbad for using the mineral waters, these waters had been in great request and many wonderful cures were attributed to them. The glauber salts extracted from them were in great demand, and they were sold by apothecaries throughout the Continent, being considered quite as efficacious as those extracted from the Carlsbad water. The people who flocked to drink the water on the spot dispensed with medical advice. It was customary for dwellers in the surrounding country to make excursions to the springs on Sundays and holidays, and to drink copiously of the Kreuzbrunnen, those who were ailing doing so in order to be cured, and those who were in good health drinking the water in order to remain well. Of the latter it may be said, as truly as Horace Walpole said of many fashionable visitors to Bath: "They went there well and returned home cured." These amateur patients and their suffering companions treated themselves in a heroic fashion. They drank from fifteen to twenty pints of the water at a time, and they took a supply home with them. At present no wise patient ventures to drink the water without consulting a physician. Dr. Kisch, one of the physicians in large practice at Marienbad, who has written an interesting work upon it, expresses his astonishment, not only that the patients in olden days should have treated themselves, which is heresy of the worst kind in a doctor's eyes, but that, despite "the irregular and irrational manner in which they used the waters, they should have been benefited in health," as is shown by the inscriptions which they left behind them in testimony of their gratitude.

From the time that Dr. Nehr took a personal interest in Marienbad the old custom of drinking the water at haphazard gradually gave place to the existing practice, when everything is done according to rule and under strict medical supervision. The Abbot of Tepel Abbey countenanced and helped him. The spring called the Ambrosiusbrunnen is named after this worthy abbot, whose name was Ambrosius Schmid. Many persons, misreading the name of the spring as Ambrosiabrunnen, marvel, when they quaff their glasses, to find how little the water realises their conception of the drink of the gods. By erecting a house for shelter in bad weather at the Kreuzbrunnen, by enclosing it carefully, by draining the surrounding marsh, and by providing baths which were supplied from the Marienquelle, Dr. Nehr changed the face of the place and rendered it more attractive. In 1791 two dependents on the abbey were allowed to build two wooden houses in which visitors might pass the night, these two houses being the precursors of the fine stone dwellings which are characteristic of Marienbad. Father Pfrogner, the successor of Abbot Schmid, entrusted his secretary, Father Karl Reitenberger, with the task of turning the wilderness into a garden, the result being seen in the beautiful grounds which now delight all those who prefer walks through green grass and clumps of flowering shrubs to walks along stony streets. Till 1808, the place was called the Auschowitzer Bad, after a stream of that name flowing through the meadows; but in that year Abbot Pfrogner gave it the name of Marienbad, placing it under the protection of the Mother of God, who, he said, was "the most powerful patroness it could possibly have." In 1813 Dr. Nehr published an account of the place and its waters, and he gave the results of his own experience there, which had extended over thirty years. He not only recommended other people to drink the mineral water, but he set them the example by drinking it himself. He died in 1820, having been a practising physician at Marienbad for upwards of forty years. The last words which he uttered on his deathbed were words of gratitude to God for his beneficent gift to mankind of the Kreuzbrunnen water.

In 1821, the year after Dr. Nehr's death, Goethe paid his first visit to Marienbad. I stated in the chapter on Carlsbad that Goethe had been in the habit of paying frequent visits to that city since he went thither and found great benefit from the waters in 1785. He was thirty-six when he first saw Carlsbad; he was an old man of seventy-two when he went to the new watering-place which was rapidly growing in importance, and he was impelled to visit it both out of curiosity and a desire to try the effect of its healing springs. In a letter to his friend Zelter he thus describes the impression made upon him by the Marienbad of those days:

"The pleasure walk here is very charming; all others of the kind are generally disagreeable, owing to pre-existing drawbacks which have been opportunely dealt with here. The architect and landscape gardener understand their business, and are accustomed to independent work. The latter seems to possess training and experience, and does not consider how the ground looks, but how it should appear; it gives him no concern to level inequalities and fill up depressions. Moreover, I feel as if I were in the North American wilderness, where forests are cleared away in order to build a city within three years. The felled firs are hewn into posts, the quarried granite rises up as walls held together with imperfectly-set mortar. Whitewashers, plasterers, and painters from Prague and other places work together in unison and with skill in the buildings which they have undertaken to rear, the result being that everything goes on with incredible speed."

Goethe not only saw the grounds laid out and the houses built, but he was present when the first school was erected. In the year that Goethe first visited Marienbad, the use of moor baths began there. These baths were the earliest of the kind in Bohemia. Having referred to them when writing about Carlsbad and Franzensbad, I need not say more about them than to repeat that they are composed of the moor earth, of which there is an abundant supply here. After trying these baths more than once, I am unable to praise them as much as some do who have taken a course of them, and derived much pleasure and benefit. A liking for a moor bath is an acquired taste. For those who are curious to learn more about their effects than I am able to give from personal experience, I subjoin the published observations of Dr. E. Heinrich Kisch, a Professor of Medicine at the University of Prague, and a practising physician at Marienbad during the season. Dr. Kisch's work on Marienbad, of which a second edition has appeared, is one of the best on the subject which I have met with. I may add that I have condensed Dr. Kisch's remarks whilst translating them.

Having experimented with these baths and gathered from his patients what their impressions were, Dr. Kisch writes to the following effect:

"Immediately after entering the bath, which, I may observe, is a semi-liquid mass of black earth, the sensation is one of excitement, of general warmth, and difficulty of breathing, while in the case of those who are unaccustomed to such a bath, palpitation of the heart is common. After the lapse of ten minutes the excitement subsides, but the face remains flushed, and there is a sensation of warmth at the top of the head. A burning sensation pervades other parts of the body, and the skin itches. The pulse is accelerated from eight to twelve beats a minute; this increased pulsation gradually diminishes; yet, during the whole period of taking the bath, it continues to be from four to eight beats above the normal rate. Two hours after leaving the bath the pulse becomes normal. During the time one is in the bath, respiration is quickened, but this ceases half an hour after leaving it. These effects are the more marked the larger the quantity of moor earth of which the bath is composed. Another effect is to increase the bodily temperature, and this lasts for a time after leaving the bath. Some of the results are ascribed to the greater heat that can be borne in a moor bath than in one containing water alone, to the mechanical action of the material, which is that of a poultice enveloping the whole body, and also to the action on the skin, and through it of the chemical constituents of the moor earth."

A gas bath is much in favour here. It consists chiefly of carbonic acid gas, and such a bath has the great advantage that the patient does not undress in order to take it. The frequent dressing and undressing is the chief objection to the hydropathic system of treatment, and, even when a single bath has to be taken during the day, many persons dislike the trouble it involves. Lord Chesterfield told his son that he knew a man who committed suicide because he considered pulling his boots off at night and pulling them on in the morning rendered life not worth living. If such a man had been a patient at a bathing place he would have felt this even more keenly; but when one can bathe, as in a gas bath, with one's clothes on, then bathing is deprived of a serious drawback. Dr. Struve, of Dresden, who is known for his efforts to produce artificial mineral waters and for establishing the Pump-room at Brighton where they were dispensed, was one of the first to experience in his own person the curative effect of a gas bath at Marienbad, the result in his case having had the effect of popularising that form of bath. He went there in 1818 for the benefit of his health. His left leg was stiffened and painful, in consequence, as he supposed, of the inhalation of hydrocyanic acid during his chemical experiments. For ten days he had drunk the Kreuzbrunnen and bathed in the water of the Marienquelle, and had applied hot fomentations of warmed moor earth or peat without deriving any benefit, and then he resolved upon trying the external application of carbonic gas. He had to be assisted to the spot where the gas streamed forth, and he subjected the stiffened limb to its action for half an hour. He began to return, when, as he writes, "who can picture the intense joy and gratitude that overpowered me when I discovered, at every new step, that power had returned to the weakened leg, and that the uninterrupted gnawing pain had left it! I walked unassisted and with ease over places which would have been an impossibility an hour ago." After three weeks' further treatment Dr. Struve left Marienbad completely cured.

Though gas baths are to be found in many other

places than Marienbad, yet they are not so well known that a few particulars about them will be superfluous. Every 1000 volumes of the gas contain seventy-four of nitrogen and twenty-six of oxygen, the remainder being carbonic acid. The gas is led from the surface of the spring, out of which it ascends, into a wooden box, within which the patient sits, the head protruding through a hole in the hinged top, this box resembling that commonly used in vapour baths. After a few minutes' time, a pleasant sensation of warmth is felt over the body, with a slight tingling in certain parts. The pulse falls within fifteen minutes after entering the bath; it then rises and beats more rapidly than the normal rate, becoming normal again within fifteen minutes after leaving the bath. If the time be prolonged, an uneasy sensation is felt in the head, as well as general oppression and discomfort. I cannot say anything personally as to the curative effects of such a bath, but I can affirm that the sensation is an agreeable one, and that I should as gladly go through a course of gas baths as of any other I have tried by way of experiment. Both Austrian and German medical men affirm that in cases of neuralgia, of rheumatism, of gout, of imperfect circulation and of particular forms of debility in elderly persons, gas baths are found to be effective and beneficial. The other baths commonly employed here are those in which the

Marienquelle water is used; this water contains a considerable proportion of carbonic acid gas, and the bather can fancy that he is lying in a huge vessel of champagne, so great is the effervescence, and so many are the tiny bells of gas which cover his body. The ferruginous water of the Ambrosius and Carolinen springs is used for bathing as well as drinking. Russian or vapour baths, differing in no respect from similar baths elsewhere, are also provided for and prescribed to patients.

Though I have written so much about the baths here, I do not wish it to be supposed that they are the principal attractions. The water drinkers are even more numerous than the bathers. Many persons for whom bathing would not be advantageous are advised to drink the mineral water. The springs are many in number and dissimilar in character. At Carlsbad each spring resembles the other in all things save the temperature, whereas at Marienbad there are springs even stronger in purgative power than any at Carlsbad, whilst others are strongly chalybeate and strengthening. The ladies who frequent Marienbad because they wish to lose superfluous fat also wish to gain power in excess of that due to the display of their natural charms, and for such patients the physician at Marienbad has more than one string to his bow, or rather has several arrows in his quiver. The main and most marked difference between the purgative waters of Carlsbad and Marienbad is that the former issue from the ground at a high temperature, whilst the latter are cold. The active principle in both is sulphate of soda. There is double the quantity of sulphate of soda in the Kreuzbrunnen, the most noteworthy Marienbad spring, than is contained in any Carlsbad spring. Instead of giving my own opinion on the subject, let me quote what Dr. Sutro says about it, his opinion being that of a German who held a physician's diploma in England as well as in Germany, and who was highly esteemed in both for his knowledge and skill. Dr. Sutro writes in his able work on the rational employment of German waters:

"While Carlsbad acts as a more powerful solvent, and as a more penetrating and lasting stimulant on the liver, skin, and kidneys, Marienbad is the more energetic and exclusive provocator of biliary excretion and of alvine secretions, and is applicable in cases of vascular erethism or local congestion, where the former would be fraught with danger."

Dr. Löschner, who, as I wrote in the chapter on Giesshübl-Puchstein, was created a baron for his services as physician to the present Emperor of Austria, employs enthusiastic terms when referring to Marienbad, where, he says, a treasure of healing springs is to be found. There are six of note, each having its special character and value. First, there is the Ferdinandsbrunnen, which exercises great influence over the mucous membrane and its affections; second, the Kreuzbrunnen, which is an unequalled aperient; third, the Waldquelle, which cures catarrh of the bronchial tubes; fourth, the Wiesenquelle, which has all the virtues of Wildungen water; fifth, the Carolinen and Ambrosiusquelle, both of which are strong ferruginous waters; sixth, the Marienquelle, which is rich in carbonic acid gas; and there is also the adjacent moor, which yields an earth or peat of excellent quality and of marvellous efficacy.

Dr. Kisch maintains that the existence of so many curative springs renders Marienbad the best of all family watering-places, adding that here every member of a family may undergo treatment at the same time—the father being cured of constipation, gout, or rheumatism; the mother of an internal malady; the daughter of debility. It is assumed, apparently, that the son is in good health. However, Dr. Kisch is not singular in thinking that most people stand in urgent need of a course of mineral waters. Medical men in Bohemia, as well as elsewhere, regard all human beings as potential patients.

The visitors to Marienbad live better than at Franzensbad or Carlsbad, the chances of getting a good dinner being greater. In Klinger's hotel, which is one of the best in Marienbad, there is a *table d'hôte*, while the hotels in the other two watering-places do not provide any such temptation to the patient who is enjoined to live by rule, who is informed that his duty is to eat and drink as little as he can, and studiously to avoid eating and drinking what he likes the best. Dr. Kisch laments that visitors to Marienbad are growing too lax in their notions of what is wholesome, and that they indulge in rich soups, mayonnaise of salmon, and other indigestible dainties. He admits that when he began to practise there, twenty years ago, the physicians were then inclined to starve their patients, and restrict them to a diet of barley broth and stewed plums; but he fears that the tendency is now toward the opposite extreme. His own view is that moderation in all things ought to be practised, and he gives his patients the following rules for their guidance.

At breakfast they may take a cup of boiled milk, cocoa-nibs, beef-tea, or very weak coffee with a well-baked roll; but they must not take black or strong coffee, thick chocolate, tea, wine, beer, rum, or rich cakes. It may be that some patients like to drink wine, beer, or rum at breakfast; it is quite certain, however, that the English do not require to be warned against so doing. The custom prevailing at Carlsbad and Franzensbad of going to a baker's shop and buying rolls or rusks for breakfast is not recognised at Marienbad. Those who supply the coffee or chocolate supply bread also. At dinner, between twelve and two, the patients may take some plain soup, a little lean beef, a roast fowl, stewed fruit, and a light pudding. Such vegetables as French beans, green peas, and asparagus are permitted, whilst the list of meats includes beef, veal, lamb, fowls, pigeons, partridges, hares, capons, larks. Some of the kinds of meat here mentioned, such as hare, are pronounced by certain Carlsbad physicians to be almost poisonous. However, the list is long enough—indeed, it reminds me of Sydney Smith's parody on Goldsmith's well-known lines—

>   Man wants but little here below,
>   As beef, veal, mutton, pork, lamb, venison show.

Among the fish that may be eaten are pike and trout, while the lover of cooked fruit may eat stewed plums, prunes, apples, pears, cherries, peaches, or apricots.

A great many things are forbidden, of which I need specify oysters only in order to add that no one would think of going to Marienbad to eat them. It seems that certain Marienbad physicians allow their patients to eat salted herrings, and Dr. Kisch rightly protests against this; but he professes his inability to understand why strawberries should be classed among forbidden fruits. At the hour when the Germans take *Vesperbrod* and the English their five o'clock tea, Dr. Kisch counsels his patients to end their meals for the day by eating a roll and drinking boiled milk, cocoa-nibs, or weak coffee; he considers supper a mistake; if indulged in, he says that it should be confined to a piece of tender meat, a soft-boiled egg, or a trout. No other drink except pure water is recommended at dinner, though in exceptional cases a little beer or light wine may be drunk. My own observation leads me to conclude that the majority of the patients at Marienbad must have received special permission to drink wine at dinner.

The physicians at Bohemian watering-places concern themselves about the time and manner in which their patients should sleep. They all advise going early to bed and getting up early in the morning, but they differ as to the propriety of taking a nap during the day. At Carlsbad and Franzensbad, sleeping by day is pronounced highly injurious, and those who give way to that weakness are strongly censured. But Dr. Kisch permits his patients at Marienbad to take a nap after dinner if they are elderly and have been accustomed to do so, and he even allows those who are very delicate and cannot sleep at night to take forty winks between breakfast and dinner. He wisely declines to lay down a general rule as to how long they should remain in bed, seeing that delicate persons require more repose than stout and full-blooded ones. He considers that seven hours are enough for most persons, and he advises his patients to go to bed at ten, and get up at five. It seems that Marienbad is frequented by enthusiasts who think they cannot drink too much of the Kreuzbrunnen, and who are in the habit of getting up to drink it at four in the morning. Dr. Kisch rightly condemns this mild form of insanity. He also warns those visitors to Marienbad who are too stout, against pursuing the Banting system, or living exclusively on milk while under treatment there. He thinks that any one desirous of losing flesh at the hazard of his health can do so most surely by uncompromising starvation.

As changes in the temperature are sudden at Marienbad, the patients there are advised to clothe themselves warmly. The ladies are least ready to follow the doctor's orders in the matter of dress, though in other matters they are most obedient. In order to overcome their reluctance to dress sensibly, it has been seriously proposed that they should not be allowed to begin the treatment unless they wore a prescribed uniform. Dr. Kisch carefully guards himself against approving of a proposition which had the support of his professional brethren, yet he admits that one of his most painful duties consists in lecturing his lady patients upon their follies in dressing. He earnestly inculcates upon them the truth that the surest way to fascinate is to become perfectly healthy.

I said at the outset of this chapter that stout ladies abounded at Marienbad, and I should add that they are kept in countenance by florid and portly gentlemen. It is noteworthy that the stout persons of both sexes are most energetic in their movements, walking hard, as well as drinking and bathing, in order to get rid of oppressive fat. Their ruddy faces, and their general air of robust health, belie the notion that they are invalids; no invalids long more keenly for good appetites than they do for bad ones. They usually leave Marienbad with lighter hearts and bodies, but they soon grow sad again at the increase in their weights. After one has been here for a few days, the array of stout persons does not appear so remarkable as at first. One becomes accustomed to the spectacle. The result recalled to my mind what I felt after seeing the giant trees of California for a time; they appeared like ordinary trees. If all the visitors to Marienbad were stout, the corpulent would attract less notice than when conspicuous among others who are the reverse. There are many slender and delicate persons who drink the iron springs of Marienbad in the hope of gaining flesh and strength.

As the houses and hotels in Marienbad are modern in construction, they are comfortably arranged. The population numbers 3000. The number of visitors during the season is about 10,000, of whom there is a sufficient proportion of English to form a small congregation in the English church, which was built in 1879. A large Roman Catholic church, in the Byzantine style, is the most conspicuous ecclesiastical edifice. To this church, which was finished in 1848, were transferred the crutches which the early visitors left behind them in the chapels in token of, and gratitude for, having been cured. There is also a German Protestant church, which King William the Fourth of Prussia helped to found, and of which his successors on the Prussian throne are the proprietors and patrons. The Jews have a Synagogue and also an hospital, wherein the poorer members of their race are carefully tended. Another hospital admits poor persons of every nationality, upwards of one hundred patients being treated there each season. There is a good theatre and a well-supplied reading-room, while there are frequent concerts and balls. The walking exercise which patients are enjoined to take can be enjoyed to perfection, the walks through the woods and up the hill-sides being many and beautiful. A favourite one is to the Hamelikaberg, where Goethe was wont to go and rest; a sandstone obelisk marks the spot where he used to sit. Nor have the memories of other persons been forgotten. A fine bronze bust of Dr. Nehr, the founder of Marienbad, stands on a pedestal of red Bohemian marble. The Abbot who did so much for the place is also honoured with a memorial in bronze; while some Poles testified in 1858 by a stone monument how thankful they felt to Dr. Karl Joseph Heidler for his services to them.

Marienbad was one of the last places which Goethe visited for the sake of the waters. Here, as elsewhere, he pursued his geological studies, and there is scarcely a rock in the neighbourhood that he did not tap with the hammer which is now preserved as a precious relic. Here, too, he fell in love with Fräulein von Löwetzow, and his poem entitled "Marienbad" was inspired by his romantic attachment. He was then seventy-four. The three seasons which he spent at Marienbad had benefited his health, the result being that he became an ardent believer in the virtues of the Kreuzbrunnen water. Several writers about Marienbad seem to have overlooked an interesting fact, which Dr. Karl Vogel, the physician who attended Goethe in his closing years, made public in 1833. This was that Goethe insisted upon drinking the Kreuzbrunnen water at home, and did so day after day and year after year between 1823, when he last visited Marienbad, till 1832, when he died. He drank upwards of four hundred bottles of that mineral water yearly. As the great poet lived till he was eighty-three, and as he did not find it necessary to revisit any Bohemian bath during the last nine years of his life, it is clear that in his case the Kreuzbrunnen water proved highly efficacious. Those visitors to Marienbad who enjoy themselves as much as Goethe did there, and derive as marked and lasting benefit from its healing springs, have good cause for regarding this beautiful Bohemian watering-place with sincere admiration, and for remembering their sojourn at it with heartfelt gratitude.

CHAPTER V.

TEPLITZ.

IT is nearly a quarter of a century since a monument was erected by the citizens of Teplitz to commemorate the eleven hundredth anniversary of its existence as a watering-place. No other Bohemian bath, and but few baths elsewhere, can boast of greater antiquity than Teplitz. When excavations were carried on several years ago, and some Roman remains were found, it was conjectured that the Romans discovered and used the mineral water here; and if this were the case, then the age of Teplitz would be even greater than is commonly supposed. However, the citizens are satisfied to date its foundation from the year 762.

A Latin inscription on a monument in the old bath-house notes the discovery of a mineral spring in 762, and mentions some of the particulars. The story is to the effect that a pig having strayed from the drove, and being followed by the swineherd, he learnt its whereabouts by hearing a loud squeal which the animal made on suddenly falling into scalding water. On reaching the spot the swineherd exclaimed, "Tepea woda," which means hot water. The proprietor of the land being informed of the discovery, he allowed his tenants to settle at the place which in the lapse of time has acquired the German name of Teplitz. There is probably as much truth in the story as there is in that of the Sprudel, at Carlsbad, having been discovered by a dog.

Of late years the references to Teplitz in the newspapers are fewer than was the case formerly. Royal and Imperial personages now prefer the baths of Gastein or Ischl to those of Teplitz, either for the sake of the water or as a place of meeting, and, though still largely frequented by invalids, Teplitz has ceased to be a regular place of resort for crowned heads. William the First of Prussia and German Emperor frequently visited it. One of his predecessors on the throne of Prussia, Frederick William the Third, went there year after year, and the citizens testified their gratitude for his patronage by erecting a monument in his honour on the Königshöhe. Another notable ruler resorted to Teplitz for the cure of ailments about which nothing certain is known. This was Peter the Great, who arrived there on the 5th of November, 1712, and who was so impatient to try the water, that he insisted upon taking a bath immediately after his arrival. Being determined that the bath-room as well as the water should be very hot, he ordered a stove to be lit in the room and heated to a high degree, whilst the water in the bath was at 110° Fahrenheit. As a further precaution against feeling chilly, he swallowed a quantity of brandy before entering the bath. It is surmised that if the Czar Peter had been less given to drinking brandy he would not have required to visit either Teplitz or Carlsbad for his health's sake. Amongst the important visitors to Teplitz who were neither Royal nor Imperial personages, were Goethe, Beethoven, and Alexander von Humboldt.

On the 1st of November, 1755, when an earthquake laid Lisbon in ruins, the principal spring in Teplitz ceased to flow for seven minutes, and then for a time it poured forth blood-red water. A century and a quarter later a more startling occurrence caused general consternation in Teplitz. There are several coalpits in the vicinity, from which immense quantities of the inferior variety of coal called lignite are extracted annually. On the afternoon of the 10th of February, 1879, the lowest workings of two of these pits were suddenly flooded, nineteen miners being drowned and 900 being thrown out of employment. Two days afterwards the citizens of Teplitz were horrified to learn that the water in the principal spring had first ceased to flow with its wonted force, had then suddenly sunk several feet, and had finally disappeared altogether. They deemed this an appalling catastrophe. The entire destruction of the city would not have been more terrible. Indeed, such a loss might be made good; houses could be rebuilt and streets remade, but to cause a mineral spring to flow again partook of the nature of a miracle. Geologists of the highest eminence, and engineers of great experience, were summoned to give their counsel in an emergency which was regarded with dismay. The citizens considered that at such a crisis in the history of Teplitz they could best manifest their feelings by abstaining from every form of amusement. Balls and private parties were abandoned, and, as a conclusive proof of the general feeling, the theatre was closed. One thing inspirited them. In Schönau, which is divided from Teplitz by a small stream, and in which the mineral waters are identical, the springs continued to flow. Yet even at Schönau, as well as in private dwellings, the springs began to fall after the lapse of a few days, and the future seemed very dark and sad.

After long and earnest consideration of the circumstances, it was resolved to make a new boring in a place not far removed from the old one, and the

I

work was vigorously prosecuted night and day. On the 12th of February the principal spring had disappeared; on the 3rd of March its source was discovered. The news not only spread through the city, but telegrams carried it to the four quarters of the globe. In Teplitz the bells from every steeple rang merry peals; the houses were adorned with flags as on days of great rejoicing; salutes of cannon and musketry were fired from the adjacent heights; the citizens pressed into the churches to return thanks to God for what they regarded as a great deliverance, and in the evening there were feasts without number, at which a telegram of congratulation from the Empress of Austria, who was then hunting in Ireland, gave especial pleasure. The Crown Prince of Austria, the Grand Duke of Baden, and the German Emperor were among the other distinguished personages who expressed their gratification at the fortunate discovery. Though the work was laborious and costly, yet it was prosecuted with so much vigour that, when the usual time in May for beginning the bathing season arrived, everything was ready, the supply of mineral water being ample and the water itself being identical with that which issued from the old outlet.

Though the anxieties which had saddened the citizens passed away when the principal spring of mineral water was rediscovered, they had to pass through a further trial of their fortitude and patience. The water had to be pumped out of the inundated coalpits in order that work in them might be resumed. These pits are upwards of five miles distant from the Teplitz springs. It was found that, as the level of the water fell in the pits, so did it at the springs; hence it was necessary to sink the springs to as low a point as that of the deepest workings in the pits. Eventually the pits were pumped dry, and the spot through which the water had broken was ascertained and the aperture closed up. Two years elapsed before the operations were completed, and then the water in the springs, both at Teplitz and Schönau, rose to its old level. Though the springs have recently fallen several feet, yet this is probably due to a preventable cause, and no fear is now entertained of an accident causing such damage or anxiety as that which has just been described.

The baths are as efficacious as ever, yet there are persons who doubt whether the mineral water is really the same as it was before the calamity of 1879. The reputation of a watering-place can be lost more rapidly than it was gained; a breath can make and unmake it. But there is no justification in fact for regarding Teplitz as less popular than in bygone days. The number of bathers is as large as before, and if it does not increase, this is attributable to the greater number of baths of a like kind elsewhere, and to their accessibility by rail. Most important of all is the circumstance that the practice does not prevail now for patients who have undergone a course of water-drinking at Carlsbad to be sent to Teplitz to undergo a course of baths.

The chief objection to Teplitz as a place of sojourn is that it has become a manufacturing place as well as one for drinking and bathing in mineral water. In many of the Bohemian valleys tall chimneys vomit forth black smoke, which forms a pall over the landscape. In Germany and Austria, manufacturers do not seem to be hindered by police regulations from polluting the air or the water. The police of both countries display great concern for the public health in certain matters, keeping sharp eyes on the meat, fish and vegetables that are sold, but they give insufficient heed to the air being kept free from smoke and the water from filth. The lignite, which is the fuel chiefly used in Bohemia, gives forth more black smoke than bituminous coal, so the necessity for consuming, or rather for preventing the formation of smoke is the greater. Certainly the quantity of dense smoke in some of these beautiful Bohemian valleys is a grievous pall over the landscape, and must be injurious to health.

The springs in Teplitz and Schönau are fourteen in number, and they do not differ from each other except as regards the temperature. The principal spring has a temperature of 120° Fahrenheit; the coldest is 76°. In the bath the water has a greenish tint, but when drawn off it is quite clear. It has neither odour nor unpleasant taste. The maladies which are benefited by bathing in this water are gout and chronic rheumatism, the results of injuries due to gunshot and other wounds, and some forms of paralysis. Why this water should prove of service in any case is as great a mystery as the curative power of some other mineral waters. Its principal ingredient is carbonate of soda; but it is quite certain that thousands who have gone to Teplitz unable to walk or move an arm have left it with entire command over their limbs. The roads to the baths are kept in good condition, so that the invalids who pass over them may not be shaken when transported in a *rollwagen*, which corresponds to the vehicle that we call a Bath chair. Some baths belong to the citizens of Teplitz, others to the inhabitants of Schönau, others to Prince Clary, and one to the Jewish community. It is common for some of the bathers to be shampooed after the bath, and it is probable that the shampooing does them nearly as much good as the bath itself. Others are made to go through a course of gymnastics. There is less rigidity in the matter of diet than at other Bohemian watering-places; instead of all patients living in the same fashion, each patient is told what will suit him best in the way of eating and drinking. Indeed, it is obvious that what would be excess in a man of plethoric habit and a martyr to gout may be quite proper for him who is paralysed in his legs or arms. The physicians at Teplitz complain, however, that their patients are apt to live too well, and that they have not the same wholesome dread of the consequences of over-indulgence in the pleasures of the table as the patients at Carlsbad. Perhaps the best proof I can give of Teplitz being still much frequented is the fact that upwards of twenty physicians and four surgeons practise there. Doctors do not congregate where patients are scarce.

Whilst the mineral water of Teplitz is chiefly employed in baths, yet it has always been drunk to some extent, and of late years its internal use has become more common. Twelve years ago special arrangements for drinking the water were made in the garden close to the Kaiser bath. When taken internally, in conjunction with the baths, the water is supposed to have a beneficial action in cases of bronchial catarrh, of excessive perspiration, of catarrh of the stomach and bladder, and of gout and rheumatism. Milk is as much relished here as mineral water. There are several " Milch-hallen," or dairies, where, at stated hours, milk can be had warm from the cow. As at Carlsbad, many of the patients drink Giesshübler water at their meals, and those who are not patients are also in the habit of drinking this pleasant table water. Two others, however, compete with it; these are Bilin and Krondorfer, the first being obtained at a place of the same name not far from Teplitz. Stronger drinks than mineral water and milk are largely consumed in Teplitz. Houses abound in which beer and wine are sold, and they are always well filled with thirsty visitors. I do not mean to imply that the persons who come here to drink and bathe in the mineral water also frequent the beer and wine shops. The truth is that a large proportion of the people in Teplitz cannot be classed among invalids, as it is a place which has been chosen as a pleasant residence by retired officers and others of small means, who desire to live comfortably and economically.

Teplitz and Schönau really form one town, the buildings between the two being continuous. Yet the two places are under separate municipalities, and in one respect the difference between them is marked. In Schönau the houses are numbered according to the system that prevails in other the treament of their brethren. It is noteworthy that a small colony of Jews settled here about 500 years ago. These Jews were the victims of many severe regulations till the time when the enlightened and tolerant Emperor Joseph the Second abolished these exceptional and tyrannical provisions, and permitted the Jews to acquire and exercise all the rights of citizenship, with the absurd exception of their being confined to a particular quarter. In Carlsbad the regulations concerning the Jews were even more stringent, no Jew being suffered to remain longer than twenty-four hours at a time; and there, as at Teplitz, they lasted till the revolution of 1848 swept away these and other bequests of a feudal past.

As I have said already, the baths of Teplitz are of special efficacy in alleviating or curing maladies which are the result of gunshot wounds and other injuries received in battle. It is a curious coincidence that Teplitz and other parts of Bohemia have been the theatre of bloody battles from the year 900 to the year 1866. In the valley where it lies, the Hussites achieved many successes and suffered great reverses, put many persons to the sword, and, in turn, were slaughtered without mercy. Teplitz was ravaged by the Swedes during the Thirty Years' War; it suffered at the hands of the Prussians under Frederick the Great. In 1813 it was the headquarters of the

Emperors of Austria and Russia and the King of Prussia, who here entered into an alliance against Bonaparte. A short journey by rail brings one to the village of Kulm, where the Allied Forces, after two days' hard fighting, gained a decisive victory over the French under Vandamme, who was taken prisoner. On the Sunday before the fight, Vandamme told his staff at dinner that they would dine at Prague the following Thursday. He dined there, as he had foretold, but he did so as a prisoner, not as a commander. Monuments on the battle-field commemorate those who fell and were buried there. Of these, the Russian one, representing a winged Goddess of Victory, is the most imposing, and the Prussian is the plainest. The Russian monument was not finished till 1836; the Prussian one dates from 1817. The Austrian monument is a pyramid, at the base of which is the Bohemian lion, and at the summit the Austrian two-headed eagle. The Russian Government paid for the first, the King of Prussia, Frederick William the Third, for the second, and the Austrian army subscribed to erect the last. The fighting in 1866 took place at a distance from Teplitz. Many Prussians who took part in it visited Teplitz the following year, in order to be cured by its waters of the injuries which they had received.

Whilst the sojourners in Teplitz can visit many

places of historical interest, they have other places to visit which possess interest of another kind. One of these is Bilin, which is a few miles distant. This is an even older place than Teplitz, its foundation dating from the year 744. It is pleasantly situated on the banks of the river Biela. The castle of Prince Lobkowitz is the most imposing object, except the rock called the Boren which, like Arthur's Seat near Edinburgh and the Rock of Gibraltar, resembles a reclining lion. The mineral springs of Bilin are a little way from the town. They are the property of the princely family of Lobkowitz, and, though they have been known for several hundred years, they have only been generally appreciated since the beginning of the present century. A large and well-appointed Curhaus has recently been erected for the accommodation of those who visit the place to drink and bathe in the mineral springs. The water is strongly alkaline, resembling that of Vichy, and having the superiority over it of being richer in carbonic acid gas. That there is a considerable demand for it is evinced by the fact of a million and a half of bottles being exported annually. Large quantities of pastilles are also prepared and exported. The water has been introduced into England, but the name is an unfortunate one, being almost inevitably mispronounced by English lips. This part of Bohemia might be called a mineral water region. Within a short compass lie three other springs of note, which are classed among what are called "bitter waters;" they are called Saidschütz, Seidlitz, and Püllna. The ordinary seidlitz powder is an imitation of the second of these three, and, in this case, the imitation is as pleasant and nearly as good as the original. Püllna water bears the closest resemblance of any Bohemian water to the German Friedrichshall and the Hungarian Bitter Water. Dr. Macpherson say that the Püllna water has been "used with great comfort" for considerable periods, without acting injuriously in any way on the system. This is consolatory, as the taste is atrocious, and the water is most powerful. The most unpleasant physic is generally pronounced the best.

The principal baths and springs in Bohemia have much in common. One of the exceptions is Königswart, which will form the subject of the next chapter. Yet there are many others which enjoy a local reputation; they number upwards of twenty in excess of those which I have described. It is possible that some of them have merits which are still unappreciated.

CHAPTER VI.

KÖNIGSWART.

Amongst the less known but not the least noteworthy of Bohemian watering-places, Königswart deserves special notice and mention. It differs from the others in many important particulars. As a rule, patients go to the others because they wish to drink or bathe in water which has a reputation for counteracting the effects of injuries received in battle, or arresting results due to eating and drinking to excess. Franzensbad is an exception, inasmuch as the patients, who belong for the most part to the gentler sex, have more in common with Venus than Mars, and have never suffered from gout. Yet there are many invalids of both sexes who require what is called tone; they suffer from debility, and their desire is to find a place where the air and the water combine to brace and strengthen their weakened chests. Königswart has been designed by Nature to meet the wants of such persons.

Königswart can be reached in half an hour from Marienbad, yet its attractions, as a watering-place, have nothing in common with the older, better known, and more frequented health resorts. What makes Königswart a most interesting place is that it differs in essential particulars from the other places to which invalids flock for relief from their ailments. The patients who visit Carlsbad have either lived too well or have been attacked by a malady from which even the most abstemious are not exempt. Those who seek relief at Franzensbad are generally women, whose lives have been rendered burdens to themselves and those nearest to them by exhausting internal maladies. At Marienbad the patients have lived even better than those who seek relief at Carlsbad, whilst the fairer patients have been cursed with premature tendency to a stoutness which gives them great discomfort, and materially lessens the admiration which they would otherwise enjoy. At Königswart, on the other hand, the victims of consumption find an amount of relief and often experience an improvement which they could not obtain elsewhere.

The mineral springs of Königswart are strengthening in an exceptional degree. They take rank with those of Pyrmont, Schwalbach, and Spa. Very little attention was paid to the mineral springs here before the year 1822. They were known to the peasants in the neighbourhood, and the one which is a sparkling water, with few chemical ingredients, was their favourite drink. In this part of Bohemia there is scarcely a village without its mineral spring, and if drinking mineral water would keep people healthy and prolong life, many inhabitants of Bohemia ought to enjoy sound health and live to a great age.

When it was found by chemical analysis that some of the springs at Königswart were rich in iron and other minerals, Prince Metternich, to whom the property belonged, determined to build houses for the reception of visitors, to erect a Curhaus and baths, and to have the place formally raised to the rank of a health resort. This was accomplished on the 19th of August, 1862, and since then the fame of the place has continued to increase. Dr. Kohn, who went to Königswart as physician to the Metternich family in 1859, and who published a small work on the place in 1873, says that in 1872 the number of patients amounted to 341, and that they came not only from Prague, Vienna, and Buda Pesth, and other Austrian and Hungarian cities, but also from Prussia and Russia, from England and France. The demand for the mineral water of Königswart at that time was so great that upwards of 4,000 bottles of the Victorsquelle were exported.

That Königswart should be a most healthy place

of abode is possible, that it should be, as Dr. Kohn calls it, an asylum for consumptives, is not equally clear. It may be true, as he says, that the health of the inhabitants is excellent. It may also be true that the proportion of those amongst them who suffer and die from chest diseases is very small. He states, and I accept his figures as accurate, that out of 385 deaths in ten years, only twenty-six are due to consumption. Yet it would be strange if a place in which the population is so small, and the conditions for longevity are so favourable, should not be singularly free from maladies which prevail in those where the pressure of population seems to lessen the limit of human life.

Writing as a critic, I should say that it would be absurd to expect to find the same diseases prevalent in Königswart which carry off thousands annually in a large capital such as Vienna. It is owing to a misunderstanding of physical conditions that certain places on the Riviera have been pronounced curative spots for those who come from large and crowded cities in England, France, and Germany. Comparatively few people die when the places are small and when every condition for prolonging life is fulfilled. At one time many patients who went to Nice for their health returned home cured. It was then a city of 20,000 inhabitants. Now the population numbers 80,000; and how many victims of consumption now recover health in Nice?

K

For this reason I doubt whether the special virtue in the air and site of Königswart has been clearly ascertained. Still, I freely admit that the situation of the place is not only most picturesque, but seems favourable to the restoration to health of those who can be benefited by bracing air and tonic waters. The chief thing in favour of Königswart is, that no other of the many Bohemian baths possesses so many advantages for the cure of maladies due to impaired nutrition and poor blood. It occupies a place amongst the Bohemian baths similar to that of Schwalbach, in Germany, and St. Moritz, in Switzerland, and the chances are very great of its fame as a health resort growing year after year. The place is very pretty; but, it must be added, it is even quieter than Giesshübl-Puchstein. The arrangements for the accommodation of visitors at Königswart are very good. This watering-place, which is the property of the Metternich family, has been the hobby and occupation of Prince Richard, the eldest son of the famous Chancellor of Austria. Visitors to it have another attraction in the castle with the fine grounds surrounding it, and the museum of curiosities contained in it. The castle is situated below the place where the springs are enclosed, and where the hotels and villas stand. The village lies between them. In the castle Prince Metternich spent the last years of his life, and he was never better pleased than when acting as guide to those who wished to see the fine collections there. The museum, though so largely increased by himself, was acquired, in the first instance, from one Huss, who had formed it. Few stories are more romantic than Huss's career, as will be seen from the brief outline which I shall give of the particulars I have collected.

Huss was born in Brüx about the middle of the last century. He belonged to a family which had supplied public executioners to Brüx and Eger. His father desired that he should become a clergyman, and wished he should be educated with that object. But the poor boy had to leave school, as the other boys would not associate with the son of the public executioner, and the schoolmaster countenanced them. At the age of fifteen, he assisted his father at an execution; two years later he was entrusted with the duty by himself; and not long afterwards he succeeded his uncle in the office of executioner at Eger. He occupied his leisure time by acting as a quack doctor; patients flocked to him. This kindled the wrath of the physicians and apothecaries in Eger, the former hating him because he deprived them of patients, the latter because his quack medicines were preferred to the drugs which they dispensed. Complaint was made to the magistrates, but they were indisposed to interfere with an officer whose services were indispensable, and one whom it would be difficult to replace.

In 1788, the Emperor Joseph the Second abolished

capital punishment, and Huss ceased to be a public functionary; not only did he lose the office of executioner but he was forbidden to practise medicine, and his quack preparations were seized and destroyed. He obeyed the letter of the prohibition, but he continued to give medical advice, though without taking a fee. It was the custom in Eger for godfathers to give presents of old coins at christenings, the result being that quantities of these coins, which had no value as currency, had accumulated in families. These coins Huss accepted as presents for his advice. As a consequence of so doing he formed a large collection of rare gold and silver coins, which was valued at 12,000 florins. The passion for collecting was aroused in his breast, and old guns, swords, armour, and other articles gradually passed into his possession. He became noted as a collector, and strangers came to see his store and to consult him about curiosities. Goethe paid him a visit and dined with him. Prince Metternich heard of Huss's collection, and expressed the desire that it should be placed in his castle at Königswart, and offered Huss a yearly pension of 300 florins if he would consent to this and act as its keeper. Huss accepted the proposal, and the citizens of Eger then thought the time had come for conferring upon him the title of honorary burgher. Thus the boy who could not receive a suitable education because he was the son of the public executioner, who had to act as executioner against his will, who lost the office through no fault of his own, had the merit of forming the museum which attracts visitors to Königswart, and he died there highly respected as its keeper.

The museum which forms a part of Prince Metternich's castle is a heterogeneous collection of curiosities. It contains specimens of the fauna and flora in the neighbourhood; coins of all kinds; specimens of paper money, including French assignats and Austrian notes between the years 1811 and 1848; the ring of Agnes Sorel; the wash-hand basin of the first Napoleon; a shoe worn by Madame Tallien; the sweetmeat box of Queen Hortense; one of the first chronometers, for which Louis XVI. paid 24,000 francs; the cap which Cavour wore indoors; Metternich's stick and snuff-box; a jewelled dagger presented to Abdel Kader by Napoleon the Third; a letter from Dumas; the manuscript of a French translation by Napoleon the Third of some lines by Schiller; an Orsini bomb; and one of the first visiting cards used by Bismarck after he was created a Prince.

It is clear, I think, that the Baths and Springs of Bohemia which I have described present many and varied attractions to those who visit them for health, and to those who do so out of curiosity. The choice of natural medicines in the form of mineral waters is very large, while the arrangements for drinking and bathing in them are very complete. In each place art has helped to embellish nature, while science has contributed to combat disease. There are many maladies which the best mineral water, taken under the advice of the most skilled physician, will not cure, yet there are few which the Bohemian mineral waters will not alleviate. What Jane Austen makes Mrs. Elton say of the waters of Bath is perfectly applicable to those of Bohemia: "When the waters do agree it is quite wonderful the relief they give." Moreover, a sojourn in the fine air and amid the charming scenery of the beautiful Bohemian valleys is itself health-giving as well as most enjoyable. Those who have once visited one of these watering-places and have derived benefit, repeat their visits in order that the improvement may be renewed or continued. It is not surprising that so many thousands should return to the baths and springs of Bohemia year after year when by so doing they are braced and inspirited anew to face the cares and to enjoy all the pleasures of life.

Yet, whether the visits are many or few, there may arise a desire in the minds of many to learn something about Bohemia in its relation to Austria. In that part of the Austrian Empire the Slavonic race is in the majority, and of late years the tendency to substitute their speech for German is very marked. The population of Bohemia is six millions in round numbers, and of these two millions are Germans in race and speech. The rivalry between the Czechs and the Germans is bitter. It is not easy for a stranger to ascertain the way in which the Government is conducted here, and the conditions under which the Bohemians exercise the Home Rule of which they are possessed. Before passing from the baths of Bohemia to describe some others in different parts of Austria, I subjoin an outline of the way in which the Government is carried on, and of the points of antagonism which divide the Bohemians into hostile political and social camps.

The Bohemian Legislature, which meets in Prague, numbers 242, and is elected by the double suffrage as in Prussia. Several members sit by virtue of their offices; some are the representatives of property and interests, and others of classes or persons. Those who sit by virtue of their offices are the Archbishop and the Bishops of Bohemia and the Rector of the University of Prague. Then the large entailed properties are represented by sixteen persons; and the large estate owners have fifty-four representatives. The city of Prague, as capital of the country, has ten, and the sixteen Chambers of Commerce have a representative apiece. Each of the sixty-two cities sends a representative, and the parishes or communes send seventy-nine. The President of the Legislative

Assembly is chosen by the Emperor, and he holds office for six years. The Assembly meets annually. It consists of a single Chamber. The electors in the last degree are a small body; they seldom exceed 150. The right to choose the electoral body is exercised by a limited number of the people, as the conditions exclude all but those who are persons of position or substance. It may be noted in passing that, while in the Kingdom of Bohemia, as in the Kingdom of Prussia, the right to choose representatives is very restricted as regards the local Parliament, the inhabitants of Bohemia, like those of Prussia, directly elect their representatives in the Imperial Parliament. If, then, wise legislation be the issue of a restricted suffrage, we should expect to find it in the Legislative Assemblies of Prussia and Bohemia. In the Prussian Parliament the most stringent, if not despotic, measures which have been passed relate to the Poles; in that of Bohemia they relate to the Germans.

I have already said that the Czechs are in a majority in Bohemia. In the Legislative Assembly there are seventy German-speaking representatives out of a total of 242. The Czech majority have used their strength like a stupid giant; the German minority, having failed to mollify them, have been driven to protesting in a striking fashion against the tyranny of their oppressors. Last December the minority formally seceded, after trying in vain to obtain a patient and considerate hearing for their demands. The elections which were held to fill up the vacant seats, had the result that, almost to a man, the seceding members were re-elected. So far from Home Rule having brought peace to Bohemia, it threatens to bring a sword. As regards the Austrian Empire, the result may prove disastrous. It is not in the nature of things that the two millions of Germans in Bohemia should quietly submit to the insults and the contumely of the Czechs. It seems clear that these Germans, while abstaining from braggadocio, are bent upon asserting and obtaining their rights. Their strength lies both in the goodness of their cause and in the moderation and firmness with which they uphold it.

Hitherto the Government at Vienna has done what it could to repress the more exorbitant claims of the Czechs. All the efforts made by the latter to induce the Emperor to be crowned King of Bohemia have signally failed. If he consented, then Bohemia would take another step in the direction of independence, and demand to be placed in the position of Hungary. Attempts have been made to interest the Hungarians in favour of the Czechs, but those have utterly failed. In the first place, the Hungarians have always fought for their own hand, and they have no sympathy or aid to spare for others; in the second, they regard the Czechs with antipathy, owing to the latter having sided with Austria against them when they drew the sword in support of their claims. It is to Russia that the Czechs look for direct countenance and efficacious support, and the real question at issue is whether the Slavs or the Teutons are to dominate in Austria. Meanwhile the Czechs have given a foretaste of what would occur on a larger scale should the preponderance of the Slavs be established and recognised. Home Rule in Bohemia has placed power in the hands of the Czechs, and they have used it to Czechify the country, if I may be allowed to coin a word for the occasion.

The Germans in Bohemia are proud of their language and their race, and whatever threatens to extirpate either, excites their apprehension and receives their bitter opposition. It so happens that the German population of Bohemia is collected together for the most part in well-defined parts of the country. In those parts German is the prevailing speech, and German ideas are predominant. Perhaps, if a criticism ought to be passed, it should take the form of the remark that in the parts of Bohemia where the Germans predominate they not only detest, but they despise the Czechs; and it is not unnatural that the majority should resent by all means at their disposal the haughty and contemptuous bearing of the minority. On the other hand, the Czech is the less educated of the two nationalities; it is not difficult to find many Czechs who cannot read or write, but a German who can do neither is almost unknown in Bohemia. Again, the menial occupations are reserved for the Czechs, who do not object to be hewers of wood and drawers of water, and who, it must be admitted, make obedient and excellent servants. Indeed, as a people, the Czechs have many lovable qualities. They are industrious and good-natured, and they are quite as sober as other Slavs.

In Bohemia, as in other parts of the world, there are men who find it an agreeable and not unprofitable trade to sow discontent and enmity broadcast. The leaders of the Czechs in Bohemia look forward to great rewards if their aspirations are realised; meantime they make agitation lucrative. Their patriotism consists, first, in labouring to place Bohemia in the position of Hungary; second, to suppress the language and literature of Germany, substituting for them those of the Czech part of Bohemia. The preservation of an ancient language is not less commendable than the preservation of national monuments; yet an old street or an old building, however picturesque, must sometimes be sacrificed in order that a modern city may expand or a family live in comfort. One cannot help regretting that the

Cornish tongue is extinct, and one cannot disapprove of preserving the poetic language of Wales; but, if Cornishmen or Welshmen were to commence a crusade in favour of the substitution of their native speech for that of England, they would be regarded as wanting in discrimination. The Czechs say that they will not speak or learn German themselves, and that they will force the Germans in Bohemia to speak and learn Czech. Thus, then, one of the phases which extreme Home Rule has assumed in Bohemia is " No German spoken here."

The Czech majority have not only legislated with a view to abolish the German language in Bohemia, but the legislation is bearing bitter fruit. Children of German parents are obliged to learn Czech if they would enter the Government service. In purely German towns, such as Carlsbad, a Czech who is temporarily residing there, has the right to insist on having an action at law tried in his own tongue, though not a single member of the Court has ever learned it. Moreover, when forty Czech labourers settle in a purely German parish, they have the right to compel a school to be provided out of the common fund for the education of their children in the Czech language. There are about 50,000 Germans in Prague, but they have no right to demand a German education for their children. Though the question at issue is largely one of language and race, the element of religion is unfortunately mixed up with it. The majority of the Czechs and Germans are Roman Catholics, but the priests have sided with the Czechs, chiefly because they find them more docile than the Germans.

The condition of things in the German districts of Bohemia having become intolerable, the manner in which the Germans were treated by the Czechs being equivalent to persecution, the German members of the Legislature made certain proposals a year ago through their leader, Dr. Schmeykal, with a view to restore harmony in Bohemia. These proposals were not even taken into consideration by the majority; they were treated with open contempt, and those who offered them were covered with opprobrium. Then the German minority resolved to retire in a body. As has already been said, their conduct has been approved by their constituents, who re-elected them with but one exception. Though re-elected, they refused to take any part in the business of the local Legislature till they received a formal and trustworthy assurance that respect would be paid to their wishes. The substance of their requirements is—first, that such an assurance shall be given by the leaders of the majority; second, that the existing regulations as regards the use of the German tongue shall be abrogated; third, that a line of demarcation shall be drawn between the Czech and German parts of the land; fourth, that the High Court of Justice, the Council of Education and of Public Worship, shall each be divided in two; and, fifth, that German shall be the tongue spoken in the Imperial Parliament. Judging from the tone of the Czech journals, there does not appear any chance of the majority yielding on one of these points. In that case the question will probably continue to cause heart-burning, and eventually a struggle on a larger scale will begin between the Teutonic and Slav elements in the Austrian Empire. The present Minister of Public Instruction, Dr. von Gautsch, has already incurred the wrath of the Czechs by refusing to assent to some of their demands concerning schools. Indeed, there are signs that the Administration of Count Taaffe, which has tacitly, if not openly, favoured the Czechs during the nine years of its existence, will now either change its course or else run the risk of an overthrow. Both the Czechs and the Germans are confident of ultimate success. They have big brothers across the frontier to whom they look for help. The Czechs regard the Great White Czar as their friend and saviour; the Germans believe that in Prince Bismarck they have a sympathiser who will never permit a people of German race and speech to be crushed with impunity. In Austria itself there are about fourteen million Germans who will side with their brethren in Bohemia. It may be that wise counsels will proceed from Vienna and be followed in Prague. Yet the contrary is quite possible; nay, it is even probable. Unless a great and salutary change occur, the result of the practical working of Home Rule in Bohemia may be a catastrophe entailing the loss to Austria of its backbone and brains as a nation in the persons of its German people.*

* The account in the last few pages on Home Rule in Bohemia elicited from the pen of Mr. E. A. Freeman a letter which appeared in *The Times* for Saturday, the 15th of October, 1887. As anything written by Mr. Freeman is read with attention and respect, I give the part of his letter which directly bears upon the subject which I have treated in the text:

"The communication in your paper of October 11 (which I saw for the first time here yesterday) headed 'Home Rule in Bohemia,' brings me back to the same position which I maintained a little time ago with regard to the use of the words 'Home Rule' as applied to Hungary and to Croatia. The relations between Hungary and Austria can teach us nothing as to Home Rule, because Hungary is an independent kingdom, Austria an independent duchy, neither of them dependent upon the other, but both joined together on such terms as the two States hold to be for their common benefit. In such a case there is no room for Home Rule, a relation which, if it has any meaning at all, means something granted or allowed to a dependency. But the relation of Home Rule does apply to Hungary and Croatia, because Croatia is a dependency of Hungary. Your correspondent starts the question of 'Home Rule in Bohemia.' Here again the phrase does not apply; at least it ought not to apply. For the kingdom of Bohemia is certainly not a dependency of the Archduchy of Austria. Both were sovereign States, *minus* their relation to the Empire; that is, since the Empire ceased to exist, both are independent States. It is open to Bohemia and

Austria, as to Hungary and Austria, to unite on any terms that they may think good; but there cannot be Home Rule in Bohemia, an independent kingdom, as there can be and is in the dependent kingdom of Croatia. Your correspondent mentions, without seeming to see the force of his own sayings, the efforts of the Bohemians to persuade their present ruler to make his rule lawful by being crowned King of Bohemia, as he has made his rule in Hungary lawful by being crowned King of Hungary. If he did so, his Bohemian subjects would perhaps no longer 'regard the Great White Czar as their friend and saviour.' Your correspondent also brings out the fact—a fact which goes further than Bohemia—that the nations which revolted against the House of Austria nearly forty years back are those which now enjoy the favours of its head, while those nations which brought that head back to power are precisely those whose demands are not granted. These points, started by your correspondent, are worth thinking over. Some of us have been thinking them over for a good many years."

CHAPTER VII.

BADEN AND VÖSLAU.

VERY few English and American tourists who visit Vienna think of going to Baden or Vöslau. The course they most commonly follow is to journey to the capital of Austria by way of Linz, taking the steamer at that place, and thus traversing the most picturesque part of the country through which the Danube flows. After seeing the objects of interest of which Vienna is full, and discovering, as they soon do, that, notwithstanding what is written in guide-books about Vienna being the Austrian Paris, the capital of Austria is a very different city from what the French are pleased to call the capital of the civilised world, they probably make an excursion to the Kahlenberg, enjoy the fine prospect from that commanding eminence, look with curiosity at the last resting-place of the Turks who died when besieging Vienna, and dine at the Kahlenberg restaurant.

If they do not leave Vienna for Trieste or Venice, and stop at Semmering on the way, they will probably make an excursion to the latter place, where a great feat in railway engineering has been performed, and where the scenery is splendid. They may have read that Baden is a watering-place near Vienna; but, believing that the only watering-place of that name worthy of a visit is the one with the double-barrelled name in the Grand Duchy of Baden, they do not go there. Of Vöslau they may know nothing except that the best known Austrian wine is produced there, this fact being insufficient to tempt them to make a journey thither. It is a mistake to neglect either place, and both not only deserve to be seen, but they are also places at which a pleasant sojourn might be made with advantage.

The distance from Vienna to Baden is seventeen and a half miles. Vöslau is a few miles farther off on the same line of railway, which is the Southern. It might be thought that one could easily get to Baden in twenty minutes by express; it will be found than an express takes forty minutes and an ordinary train an hour to get over the ground. Though Brighton is three times the distance from London that Baden is from Vienna, yet a Londoner can get to Brighton in almost as short a time as a Viennese, travelling by an ordinary train, can get to Baden.

What struck me on reaching Baden was the completeness of the change; it was nearly as great as that between London and Brighton. I could scarcely believe that the wonderful city of Vienna was less than eighteen miles distant. The scenery is not only that of the country, but also of a very pretty country, diversified with mountain ranges. I was struck, moreover, with the points of resemblance between this Baden and Baden-Baden, the Helenenthal in the former being not less beautiful a valley than the Lichtenthal in the other; whilst a castle perched high up on the mountain side recalled that which attracts visitors to Baden-Baden. The Schwechat, which flows through the Helenenthal, is a stream of the same size as the Oos, which flows through the Lichtenthal.

Baden is not merely a small town where there are mineral waters, and to which the Viennese resort for change of air and scene; but it is also a watering-place to which invalids flock from many parts of Europe, and where a regular course of bathing and water-drinking can be pursued under medical supervision. The visitors number 15,000 yearly, and the majority undergo a regular course of treatment. There are more than a dozen resident physicians, and it is as common to consult a doctor on arriving there as it is at other watering-places. Some of the doctors complain that invalids venture to treat themselves. These foolish persons are styled "savages." The doctors comfort themselves with the reflection that the "savages" will take the wrong baths, drink mineral water in an unorthodox style, and suffer well-deserved torments. It may interest many persons to learn that Baden was a favourite place of resort for Mozart and Beethoven, and that both composed there several of their finest works. The greater part of Beethoven's Ninth Symphony was composed in Baden. Grillparzer, the poet of whom the Austrians are justly proud, was a frequenter of this place. A monument to him has been erected here.

The literature relating to Baden is extensive. Out of the books written about it, the most useful appear to be two by medical men, Dr. Hoffmann and Dr. Schwarz, who have practised in Baden for many years. The work by Dr. Hoffmann was published in 1882, and that by Dr. Schwarz appeared last year. To both I am indebted for many interesting particulars.

It is noteworthy that Baden is a watering-place of great antiquity. The mineral springs which abound may have flowed in prehistoric times. They were known to the Romans as *Aquæ Pannonicæ*. Thirteen years before Christ, the Roman army under

Augustus overspread this part of the world, fought against and conquered the Wends, a Celtic race that occupied it, and took possession of the town, which they called Vindobona, and which is now known as Vienna. It is believed that the mineral waters of Baden were employed by the aborigines whom the Romans subdued, and there is no doubt that the Romans themselves made use of them. In the "Itinerary" of the Emperor Marcus Aurelius it is noted that the road from Vindobona (now Vienna) to Scarbantia (now Oedenburg) passes Aquis. This place is the same distance from Vindobona that Baden is from Vienna. Moreover, remains have been found at Baden showing that companies of the X., XIV., and XXX. Legions halted here on their way to or from Vindobona, and that a Roman bath stood near the spot where the principal mineral spring issues from the ground.

For centuries after the Roman power had declined, this part of Europe was a battle-ground. It is not till the year 1173 that any mention of this Baden is found in writing. In that year the Margravine Agnes of Tulln presented two vineyards near Baden to the convent of Klein-Mariazell, and in the deed of gift the locality is described as being that which is called Baden in our tongue and bath in Latin—"*In loco qui lingua nostra dicitur Baden, Latinè vero balneum.*" As early as the middle of the eleventh century a church was built there; another church and a monastery were built in the thirteenth. A Margrave of the Paden family had built a castle on the site, probably, of the present school-house. Franz Haag, the chief of a robber band from Bohemia, took forcible possession of this castle. By command of the Emperor Frederick the Third the place was besieged and recaptured, and the robbers and their leaders were hanged behind Mount Calvary, which still bears the name among the people of " Gallows Mountain." This spot long continued to be the Tyburn of Baden, and the saying is current that " the highest gibbet in the land is to be found there."

In 1466, Baden had become so important as to receive the privilege of being a market town and being fortified; soon afterwards, however, it was destroyed and the surrounding country devastated by the Hungarians under Matthias Corvinus. This was not the first time that the Hungarians had overspread and wasted the country. Had it not been that the Emperor Frederick the Fourth conferred special privileges upon Baden, allowing its inhabitants to levy tolls and elect a council, it might not have risen from its ashes. After it was rebuilt and refortified, the ruthless Matthias Corvinus and his fierce followers again attacked, plundered, sacked, and burnt it to the ground. Half a century later, when the town was flourishing again, the Turks appeared and emulated the Hungarians as destroyers. This was in 1529; in 1683 the Turks reappeared, slaughtered such of the inhabitants as did not escape to the mountains, and set fire to the houses. When the Turks had departed, the surviving inhabitants begged people from the surrounding country to come and help them to rebuild the town and settle in it. Owing to the damage then wrought by the Turks, few documents have been preserved about Baden's early history. The plague raged here during the years 1613, 1644, and 1691. It broke out in other parts of Austria in 1713, and carried off many persons in Vienna, but not a case then occurred in Baden. Though fires were frequent, the place flourished and the inhabitants grew rich. For this they had chiefly to thank the mineral springs, which attracted many persons to their town.

The earthquake which destroyed Lisbon in 1755 was felt at Baden. The springs underwent several changes; the principal one lost its clearness, and for a considerable time its water was mixed with red sand, whilst the quantity of gas contained in it was largely increased. Moreover, the water has continued since then to be richer in gas than it was before. A further result of the earthquake was the bursting forth of the spring which now supplies water to the Angel's Bath. Towards the end of the last century, the place grew so rapidly that the old fortifications had to be pulled down to make room for houses.

Shortly after the beginning of the present century, the visitation of a foreign foe partially reminded the people of what their forefathers had felt when in the hands of the Hungarians and the Turks; but the French, who invaded Austria in 1805 and 1809, were more merciful than previous conquerors, levying tribute, but sparing lives and property at Baden. Fire was as great a terror to the town as a foreign enemy; at intervals many houses had been burnt down, but in 1812 as many as 125 were laid in ashes at once, and many of the inhabitants were reduced to absolute beggary. This fire, which was the last as well as the most disastrous, proved to be of benefit to the town, seeing that the houses were rebuilt on a better plan; and it is due to this cause, in no small measure, that the houses, streets, and gardens as they appear to-day are so well arranged and laid out. From the year 1812 till now, Baden has continued to increase and prosper. Its recent history is a record of the erection of new bath-houses, of public and private buildings. The year 1866, which was a dark one for Austria in general, was a bright one for Baden, as then it was first lit up with gas.

The Cetisch range of mountains, on the southern slope of which Baden lies at the height of about 700 feet above the sea, shelters it from the north and north-east winds. The temperature is neither very high in summer nor very low in winter. In spring and autumn the weather is raw and cold. The mean temperature for the year is 50° Fahrenheit. Thus Baden is a pleasanter place of residence, as far as climate goes, than the capital of the Austrian Empire, and many wealthy Viennese have villas here, which they occupy during several months in the year. The locality resembles a huge park dotted with villas. Vines grow all around, and the wine made from the grapes which they yield is excellent when pure. But pure Austrian wine is as difficult to procure as pure claret. Hungarian wines are much cheaper as well as stronger than the Austrian, and they are largely used for blending with those prepared in this neighbourhood. Yet some of the wine-growers retail their produce, and one can easily find out where to get a glass of unadulterated wine. A branch of fir projecting from the door denotes that new wine may be had within; a bunch of straw denotes that old wine is procurable; and if a piece of red cloth be displayed along with the branch of fir or bunch of straw, the passer-by knows that red wine is sold there. The inhabitants are German by race, and they speak the Viennese dialect. Dr. Hoffmann laments that the manners and customs of the capital have somewhat corrupted the innocent natives of Baden. He considers them less grasping than the inhabitants of other watering-places, yet he admits that they have keen eyes for the main chance, and are active in making hay whilst the season lasts.

Owing to the equable and moderate temperature, plants and flowers of all kinds are luxuriant. As springs of warm water abound, the earth is never very cold, and this contributes to the growth of almond and fig trees, and of plants which generally come to perfection in more southerly spots. Higher up on the mountains the flora has an Alpine character. Large game abound in the woods. Vermin, such as foxes and badgers, are almost as plentiful as deer. On the grassy slopes there is good grazing ground for cattle, sheep, and goats. All kinds of vegetables grow well in the gardens. Besides grapes, the fruit is excellent, and the plums, apples, and pears find a ready market in Vienna. Pine and beech trees clothe the mountain slopes; the former impart fragrance to the air.

Thirteen mineral springs are in use, and all resemble each other in their constituent parts, the chief of which is sulphur. Wherever a hole is bored mineral water is found. Even in the bed of the Schwechat stream, mineral water bubbles out. The water contains salt as well as sulphur, and the predominant gas is sulphuretted hydrogen. After drinking the mineral water I can confirm Dr. Hoffmann's statement that it has a very unpleasant salt taste and smells of rotten eggs. Some ladies who bathe in it are unpleasantly reminded of the nature of its ingredients when they find the metallic cosmetics with which they have beautified their skins suddenly change to a dark brown or jet black. All ladies are warned against employing such cosmetics, and, when they find that the consequences are serious, they gladly obey. They are also warned against wearing gold or silver ornaments when they go to bathe, as the gold acquires the hue of copper and the silver of iron. In answer to those who contend that the presence of sulphuretted hydrogen in the water may prove injurious, Dr. Schwarz replies that the quantity is just sufficient to do good, and not enough to work mischief. Dr. Hoffmann's decision is that, should the sulphuretted hydrogen really act injuriously, the salt in the water forms an antidote. It may comfort timid persons that the antidote accompanies the poison.

The mineral water is more used for bathing than for drinking purposes. When issuing from the ground its temperature ranges from 80° to 95° Fahrenheit. There are sixteen well-appointed bath-houses. One of them the Caroline bath, is specially set apart for ladies; but Dr. Hoffmann notes that most ladies prefer going to the bath where gentlemen bathe also. The truth is that the custom prevails of bathing in common. A dress is worn by both sexes, and as the bathers remain immersed up to their chins, all that the spectator sees is a mass of more or less unattractive heads. It is said that each bath is completely emptied and cleansed every Friday, and this is held forth as a recommendation. I should enter the bath with still greater pleasure if I were assured that the water was renewed every day.

A long list of ailments is given for which these mineral waters are recommended. The principal ones are rheumatism, anæmia, gout, and scrofula. A large number of the poorer Viennese, particularly children, suffer from anæmia and scrofula, and a course of treatment at Baden is of great service to them. Hospitals and asylums have been founded for the reception and treatment of the poor; thus Baden is a great benefit to Vienna as well as a pleasant place of resort. I have been informed that in many cases the waters have an unpleasant action when first employed. Those who come with coughs begin to cough oftener after using them. Gouty and rheumatic patients become weaker and uncomfortable after bathing for a fortnight. Most patients appear to regard these results as natural, and when they suffer from fresh pains they consider that they are in a fair way towards recovery. "The pains have begun" is an exclamation which it seems to please them to make. By common consent among the patients the cure is supposed to last either twenty-one or forty-one days. The doctors protest against this, and say, with justice, that the number of baths to be taken must be determined by the patient's condition; but they find it hard to fight against a general and deeply-rooted opinion.

Patients are subjected to a regular course of dietary, and this, combined with the fine air, may contribute as much to their cure as the baths and waters. A long list of things to be avoided is given; but this I need not reproduce, as it greatly resembles lists which I have given in previous chapters. The doctors at Baden take good care that their patients shall not go wrong for lack of minute advice. Thus they are warned to clothe themselves warmly and carefully to avoid catching cold. They are told not to walk too fast, and not to fatigue themselves. They are told also, what they might find out for themselves, that it is well to remain indoors during bad weather. Should the weather be fine, they need not lack amusement. As at other watering-places, a band plays several times a day. There is a good theatre, and it is quite possible to go to the theatre in Vienna and return in time for bed. One of the newest attractions is a Curhaus, which is as fine a building of the kind as I have ever seen. A restaurant which forms part of it is well conducted, and a dinner there is most enjoyable. The Curhaus stands in the park, which is extensive, which has alleys of trees and beds of flowers, and is a place wherein one can sit or walk for the greater part of the day. When seated on the terrace at the restaurant one is reminded of the terrace behind the Curhaus at Homburg, and one can with difficulty realise that so large a city as Vienna is near at hand.

Vöslau is distant from Baden an hour by road and ten minutes by rail. Though much the smaller place of the two, it is not the less beautiful. The mineral waters belong to the category styled "indifferent," yet this does not imply that they are inactive. The waters of Schlangenbad, in Nassau, are "indifferent" also; they have a high repute, however, for their curative properties. The regular use of the Vöslau waters did not begin till 1822, though long before they had been used and prized by the country people. As the spring, after issuing from the ground, flows with a strong current, it was employed at one time to drive a mill, and it was known as the warm brook. On the 27th of February, 1768, an earthquake occurred at Vöslau, and affected the mineral spring by raising its height and increasing its temperature. At present the temperature is 75° Fahrenheit. A notable fact in the annals of Vöslau is that an apothecary's shop was first opened there in 1862. This was consequent upon the increase of visitors coming to be cured. Whereever visitors congregate there is a demand for drugs. It is only in remote country places that people manage to live and die comfortably without the aid of medicine.

The rising popularity of Vöslau as a health resort is proved by the increasing number of visitors to it since medical men began to send patients. In 1853 the number of visitors was 1183; last year it was upwards of 4000, and this does not include those who come from Vienna on a pleasure trip. At Gainfarn, a short distance from Vöslau, there is a hydropathic establishment under the charge of a resident physician, and this is, too, an attraction. The air is very light and pure at Vöslau, so that what the Germans style an "air cure" can be enjoyed. Another form of cure is drinking whey made from the milk of cows or sheep. Both here and at Baden the grape cure is prosecuted in the autumn. The grapes are very fine and very cheap. I enjoyed the Vöslau grapes; but then I ate them for pleasure, not as medicine, and I doubt whether they would not soon pall if I had to swallow several pounds of them daily for several weeks. I have heard that some physicians order as many as from six to eight pounds of grapes to be eaten every day by their patients. This seems to me far too much of a good thing. Those who steadily follow this form of cure lose all relish for grapes. The patients are enjoined to abstain from eating much else, and to dine and sup off fish, fowl, game, and light puddings. They can do this the more easily, as they have neither appetite nor room for heavy food.

It is in favour of the mineral waters of Vöslau that they are not said to cure everything, the maladies being limited in number for which they are supposed to act beneficially. Hysterical and neuralgic disorders, debility, and indigestion are the principal ailments which are relieved or cured here; and I am told it is because so many actual cures are effected that the fame of Vöslau as a watering-place spreads wider every year. Dr. Friedmann, who has practised here many years, writes strongly in praise of the baths. Those who suffer from loss of appetite would do well to visit Vöslau, as one marked result of a bath is to create a longing for food. Delicate and nervous children are especially benefited by the Vöslau waters. The usual amusements are provided; concerts, balls, and plays being given in the Curhaus. The walks and drives are many, and the walks through the balsamic pine woods close at hand contribute to restore health and strength to the sufferers from delicate chests.

Both Baden and Vöslau are visited by some patients who have taken a course of waters at Carlsbad or Marienbad, and who, after drinking the Sprudel or Kreuzbrunnen for several weeks, require an "after-cure" in the form of repose and refreshment. I have not heard of any English and American visitors to Carlsbad or Marienbad trying Vöslau or Baden for an "after-cure;" many of them go to the Tyrol, where they follow the grape cure; but they might find it a pleasant change to try the watering-places near Vienna.

The Viennese are to be congratulated upon having such charming watering-places so near their city. They seem to appreciate the advantages which they enjoy, and they gladly sing the praises of Baden and Vöslau. I cannot say that their admiration for them is undeserved or exaggerated. But I must note a blot on the landscape, or rather, perhaps, a dark cloud in the sky. Looking from the mountain slopes behind Baden upon the rich and wide plain wherein Vienna stands, one sees countless tall chimneys from which volumes of smoke issue. The air is obscured and contaminated. I remarked this to my Viennese friends, and they quite agreed with me in deprecating the spectacle. I suggested that the police authorities should take steps for abating the nuisance. They replied that in Austria the police think more about politics than the public health. I told them what Palmerston did during the time that he presided over the Home Office, when he proved himself to be as efficient a Home Secretary as he had been brilliant as a Foreign Minister. They did not know, and they were interested to learn, that Palmerston had succeeded in persuading Parliament to pass an Act which has nearly freed some parts of London from the pest of smoke. May I express the hope that some other energetic Home Secretary, by completing Palmerston's work, may immortalise his name ? My friends further told me that if smoke were a Social Democrat, it would not long pollute Austrian air. I said to them that it was nearly as bad; that it was quite as much to be dreaded as the Turks when they besieged their city; and that it was as easy to compel manufacturers to prevent the smoke being formed in their furnaces as it was to repel the onslaught of the Turks. I trust that the Viennese police may yet turn their attention to the smoke question. They will doubtless do so, and act with energy once they are convinced that the smoke which spoils the prospect and pollutes the air around Vienna is quite as noxious as the most rabid utterances of the wildest Anarchist.

CHAPTER VIII.

ISCHL.

NATURE has provided Ischl with a lovely site, and the presence there of notable personages has rendered it famous. It is a favourite resort of crowned heads and a meeting-place of great statesmen. The statesmen of Germany, Austria, and Russia have assembled there either to compare notes, plan policies, cement friendships, or simply to recruit their healths. Ischl has been the summer residence of the Empress of Austria since 1860, while the Emperor has also been a frequent visitor, as well as the Crown Prince. The Austrian Imperial family have made Ischl fashionable.

An interesting article might be written concerning the effect of Royal personages taking up their abodes at given spots. The presence of George the Third, and long afterwards of Queen Adelaide, at Weymouth largely helped to bring that watering-place into repute. The small fishing village of Brighthelmstone was gradually converted into the large and lively town of Brighton, after George the Fourth took a fancy to live there. Few tourists go to Balmoral, and still fewer attend church on Sunday in the absence of the Queen. In England and Scotland vulgar curiosity induces many persons to mob a crowned head, and it is not the highest class which dogs the footsteps of Royalty. But in Austria the aristocracy consider it a duty to follow when the Sovereign points the way, and thus the place wherein the Empress or the Emperor delights to dwell is largely frequented by the nobility. This has a good and a bad result. The good result consists in the small mountain village being renovated and cleansed, in the removal of nuisances, and the embellishment of its houses and streets. An enormous rise in prices is the bad result, though for this there is a compensation in the circumstance that the pleasure-seekers who infest cheap places and render them unendurable are deterred from coming very often or remaining very long.

Yet a health resort does not flourish if it have nothing else than the presence of Royalty to recommend it. Those who set the fashions like variety, whether it take the form of change in apparel or change of scene. There are solid reasons for the reputation which Ischl enjoys, and the credit of discovering them is due to Dr. Wirer. His service to

Ischl is equivalent to that of Dr. Becher to Carlsbad Dr. Adler to Franzensbad, and Dr. Nehr to Marienbad. Dr. Wirer discovered the advantages with which nature had endowed Ischl; he made them known to the members of his own profession; he convinced his medical colleagues, after convincing himself, that his views were sound and his conclusions right, and the suffering public took the advice of his colleagues and himself, and visited it in order to be healed. Many years before a crowned head made Ischl a place of sojourn, it had become noted for the cures wrought there. The presence of Royalty supplied but an outward and visible proof that the place was attractive and important.

Dr. Wirer visited this part of the world about 1820, and he was struck with Ischl on account of the mildness and equability of its climate; he was likewise struck with the curative effects of its brine baths upon the patients to whom he prescribed them. He laboured to convert it into a health resort, and his efforts were so far successful that in 1822 a suitable house where brine could be used in baths was erected, this bath-house being the first of the kind in Austria. He succeeded in effecting arrangements for providing whey, drinking whey being considered a good adjunct to bathing in the salt water. Two members of the Austrian Imperial family, the Archduke Francis

Charles and his wife, took a liking to Ischl, spent much time there, and actively aided Dr. Wirer in his endeavours to beautify it. When they died, in 1878, a drinking fountain, which is really a work of art, was erected as a memorial of them.

The earliest improvements in Ischl consisted in pulling down the primitive and unsanitary houses and erecting better and healthier ones, in making new streets and laying out gardens. Dr. Wirer died in 1843. Many years before his death his practice had grown so large that he was enabled to save much money. He bequeathed the larger part of his fortune to founding an institution wherein poor patients may obtain medical advice and treatment. Moreover, the sum of money which he left behind him contributed to build a new bath-house, a swimming bath, and the esplanade on the left bank of the river Traun, which is the regular and agreeable lounging-place for visitors. A colossal bust of Dr. Wirer in bronze, bearing the inscription, "Grateful Ischl to its benefactor," commemorates his life and labours here. Dr. Pollak, who settled in Ischl at the request of Dr. Wirer, wrote about it in a way which attracted notice, and Dr. Mastalier emulated Dr. Wirer in leaving a part of his savings to continue the work which was begun through Dr. Wirer's generosity. Dr. Kaan, who has practised in Ischl for a long period, and whose work relating to it I have found the most useful of all the German ones on the subject, says with apparent justice that Ischl is greatly indebted to its doctors. Happily, perhaps, there is no lack of them. There are ten hotels and twelve doctors in Ischl.

Dr. Kaan writes about Ischl not only with practical knowledge and experience, but with warm enthusiasm. He tells the reader in the preface to his work that he had practised his profession at St. Petersburg, Meran, and Innsbruck, before settling here. He complains bitterly that the place is undervalued and decried by his fellow-countrymen who contribute to the newspapers of Vienna. These journalists, to whom he attaches opprobrious epithets, are said to be fond of praising Reichenhall, in Bavaria, and giving it the preference over Ischl, and to prefer going to Switzerland, and urging others to do likewise, instead of enjoying and magnifying the charms of the Salzkammergut and the Tyrol. How far these complaints are well founded I cannot tell. But I have found Ischl very different from any place in Switzerland, and quite as worthy of a visit as any other health resort. I think, too, that the general public is of my opinion. In the height of the season it is difficult to get a bed, and though the season was approaching a close during the time of my visit, the esplanade was by no means deserted. If, as Dr.

Kaan complains, the Viennese journalists have striven to give Ischl a bad name, they have signally failed in rendering it unpopular.

The purposes for which patients visit Ischl are twofold. They hope to benefit by its genial and equable climate as well as by the brine baths; the air is regarded as quite as curative as any mineral waters. Indeed, the mineral waters at Ischl are not remarkable. One spring, named after Dr. Wirer, on the right bank of the Traun and in the part of the town which is called "Gries," gives forth very cold water which is so slightly mineralised as to have no perceptible taste. Another spring, called Maria Louisa, is two miles and a half distant from the town on the Salzburg road, which runs along the right bank of the river Ischl. This yields a weak saline water, which is not drunk on the spot, but is bottled and dispensed in the room at the principal bath-house where other mineral waters are supplied. A cold sulphur spring is used for bathing purposes. More importance is attached to the brine baths. The brine is obtained from the rock salt in the mountains. Pipes containing ordinary water are carried to the deposits of rock salt. When the water is saturated it is reconveyed to the salt-works, and there yields 26 per cent. of salt. The brine baths here resemble those which can be had at Reichenhall, Nauheim, and Kreutznach in Germany, and at Droitwich in England. They do not differ materially from hot sea-water baths. To prevent misapprehension I should add, perhaps, that in translating the German *Soolbad* into brine bath, I do not mean to convey that persons bathe in the concentrated brine. The truth is that a certain portion of the brine—about three parts in twelve for an adult—is mixed with ordinary water, and a very strong salt-water bath is thus formed. Baths are provided in which other substances are used, such as the extract of fir needles or of moor-earth. The brine is also applied to the throat and air passages in the form of spray, and very good results are said to be produced by inhaling it. There is a hydropathic establishment here, where the well-known processes of applying cold water are conducted under the direction of a medical man. There is a large swimming bath and "wave baths," the latter being an attempt to represent artificially the action of the waves of the sea. The spoiled daughters of luxury who are very rich and have very sensitive skins, indulge in whey baths. Such baths are supposed to calm the nervous system; but their use may be chiefly due to the fact that they render the skin soft to the touch and silky in appearance.

A common complaint at many watering-places on the Continent is that persons go and drink the mineral waters, and take baths, without consulting a doctor. There is no restriction at Ischl upon water-drinking; indeed, the mineral water has no attraction; but bathing cannot be carried on there except under medical sanction. The keeper of the bathing establishment is forbidden under penalty to sell tickets for brine baths to any one who is not provided with a doctor's permit. Hence, the patients are obliged to get medical advice before beginning their "cure." At some Italian watering-places a visit to the official doctor is compulsory; but one visit and the payment of ten lire restore freedom of action to the patient; he needs not return to the doctor unless he think fit, and he may drink as much mineral water as he pleases and bathe as often as he chooses to pay for a bath. Sometimes the regulations about medical permission give rise to puzzling questions. I revisited Franzensbad some time ago. Wishing to take a bath, I found that I could not do so as it was after 3 p.m., the hour at which the bathing-houses are closed. Finding the gas bath-house open, and being curious to try the effect of a carbonic acid gas bath, I went and had one. That bath has the convenience of not requiring undressing. Beyond a sensation of warmth all over the body, I did not find any marked result from it. I was not called upon to pay till I was leaving, and then I was asked for the name of the medical man who had prescribed the bath, in addition to my own name and address, the object being to enter these particulars in a book. When I told the woman who kept the book that I had taken the bath as an experiment, and also because I could not get any other, she was sorely perplexed, and informed me that it was contrary to the regulations. She said that she hoped no harm would ensue, but she evidently feared lest something dreadful would occur. Happily, I was none the worse, and I trust that she did not suffer either.

Now, though no one is allowed to inhale brine or bathe in it at Ischl without a doctor's prescription, any one may take a Russian vapour bath there by paying the price. To take such a bath is a greater risk for some persons than bathing in salt water is for anybody. I found the Russian bath comfortable, and the attendant thoroughly competent. Every reader may be assumed to be acquainted with a Turkish bath. The efforts of the late Mr. Urquhart to popularise these baths in England have been as successful as he could have desired. It may not be superfluous, however, to observe that the name Turkish bath is a misnomer, the proper name being Roman or hot-air bath. The sweating baths in which Mahomedans delight vary in different places; those of Morocco, Egypt, and Turkey being dissimilar in matters of detail; yet a real Turkish bath more closely resembles what is commonly styled a Russian bath than the bath which is known in England and America as Turkish.

In the Russian bath the active agent is hot steam, and the soothing effect on the air passages of the warm, moist vapour is both striking and curative. Such a bath differs from the vapour baths in use at English hydropathic establishments in this respect— that in it the steam is inhaled, whereas in them the steam is merely an agent for producing perspiration, the head being left uncovered by the waterproof which confines the steam round the rest of the body. Inhaling the steam is half the cure in a Russian bath. It is to produce a like result that a "bronchitis kettle" is used in a bed-room by those who suffer from an irritated throat and chest; but, if a Russian bath were taken, double the good effect would be produced. The introducer of a well-appointed Russian bath into London would be a far greater benefactor than Mr. Urquhart, to whom Londoners are indebted for the so-called Turkish baths. At Marienbad and other places on the European Continent this form of bath bears the name of the "Irish bath." In olden days the Irish were in the habit of taking baths in the same way that Russian peasants do now. If the Irish bath, in its improved form, were introduced into

England by some energetic Irishmen, the Saxons might accept the boon with gratitude.

In addition to taking baths of various kinds and drinking mineral water, the patients at Ischl have other forms of cure at their command. Chief among them is the whey cure, to which reference has already been made, and which is pursued methodically here. Professor Seegen, one of the highest authorities on health resorts and methods of cure, pronounces Ischl to be specially adapted for the whey cure, the climate admirably suiting the patient for whom such a kind of treatment is appropriate. The whey used is made from the milk of cows, sheep, or goats. It is supplied at the pump-room, and patients go thither as early as six in the morning to drink it. Whilst the effect of drinking whey may be beneficial, the taste of it is most disagreeable, the strongest sulphurous mineral water not being more nauseous. Another form of cure consists in drinking butter-milk. This is far more palatable than whey. For affections of the chest whey is prescribed, and butter-milk for certain diseases of the stomach. A form of treament in use here is intended to purify the blood, and it can be pursued only in the spring and early summer; it consists in eating plentifully of Alpine strawberries. Few patients object to follow it.

The great charm of Ischl for those who are not

invalids is its situation. It is in the heart of the Salzkammergut, at an elevation of 1600 feet above the level of the sea. It lies at the confluence of the rivers Ischl and Traun. Mountains rise and wide valleys open up on all sides. Each walk and prospect seems more beautiful than the other. At convenient distances are the lakes which form the charms of the Austrian Alps, such as the Traun lake, the Atter lake, the Mond lake, the Hallstädter lake, and the Wolfgang lake. A favourite excursion is to the salt mines, which can be reached in an hour. Permission to visit them is easily obtained, and the payment of a few florins will ensure the illumination of some of the more curious parts. I was satisfied to read about them, and can believe that the spectacle of the lights playing on the rock salt is a fairy one. But I have descended as many mines and entered as many caves as I care to do. The taste for entering caves, which is widespread and strongly developed, might be classed by an ingenious speculator among the survivals of the days when prehistoric man dwelt in them. In like manner, living in house-boats may be a survival of the fondness of primitive man for building his dwelling on piles far out in a lake. He went there to be secure against his savage fellows or wild beasts. Civilised man may live in a house-boat or a yacht to escape from the tax-gatherer.

There are mountains to climb near Ischl as well as mines to explore, and the view from any of their summits is grand. Not far up one of the mountain sides is an ice cave, which can be seen without strain or discomfort, and which is well worth a visit. There are easy and level roads for those who do not care to ascend the mountain slopes, and these roads are well kept. At every turning a fresh view of green meadow or flowing river delights the eye, and tempts the way-farer to continue his course.

In the town itself there are many well-shaded walks through gardens, in addition to the fashionable promenade along the esplanade, where is the *Café* Walter, a favourite resort of visitors. Even patients are allowed to please their tastes at meals here, the result being that they indulge in good things to an extent which must strain their digestive organs; rich cakes are eaten at breakfast instead of the simple rusks which are prescribed to patients at Carlsbad. The Curhaus is a large and handsome building, standing in a garden filled with choice flowers. In this garden there is a meteorological station, where one can see a record of the temperature and the weather all over Europe, where thermometers and barometers indicate both the heat of the air and the pressure of the atmosphere, and a sundial shows the time of day. It is contemplated to lay out a part of the garden with specimens of the entire Alpine flora. Close at hand is a museum containing a variety of articles. Among them is a collection of the minerals and stones, the plants and insects of the district. A case contains Roman remains found at Hallstadt; these are chiefly metal ornaments, though among them is a piece of mosaic which probably formed part of the floor of a bath. In another case there are remains from lake dwellings in the Attar lake: these are mostly bones of animals, jawbones containing teeth predominating. A curiosity of another kind is a spinnet on which Mozart played when young; it resembles a modern grand piano in form. At present the collection is heterogeneous, but it is the nucleus of what may become a very interesting one when enlarged and classified.

Though Ischl is but young amongst watering-places, it has an old history. It formed a part of the Roman province of Noricum, and many Roman coins have been found in the neighbourhood. Quite as interesting is a tombstone of a Roman Christian which is now embedded on the south side of the church tower. The inscription is to the effect that it was erected in happy memory of Romanus by his wife, that Romanus was the son of Maternus, and that he died in his eightieth year. This might be instanced as a proof that people lived to a good old age in the Roman days. It is known that salt-works existed in the neighbourhood of Ischl as far back as the tenth century. At the middle of the sixteenth century, most of the inhabitants of the locality were Protestants. At the beginning of the seventeenth century, they were ordered to become Roman Catholics, and the troops of the Archbishop of Salzburg gave practical effect to the order by slaying those who refused to obey it. Several years elapsed before the profession of Protestantism was tolerated again. At present, out of a population of 36,000 in the Salzkammergut, 5000 only are Protestants. During the war which raged in the eign of the Empress Maria Theresa, much havoc was wrought here, while as much damage was done by the French during the first ten years of this century. In addition, the French compelled the inhabitants to pay heavy contributions. I was glad to note at the saltworks that a working man's co-operative store has been established and is thriving. I should add that similar stores exist in other parts of Austria.

I have written enough to make it clear that Ischl has many attractions. It is quite natural that the Empress of Austria should prefer it to many others as a place of abode in the summer. The Imperial residence is built in the style of a Swiss chalet. The surrounding grounds are extensive, and they are beautifully laid out. To repeat what I said at the outset of this chapter, her presence and that of other members of the

Imperial family, as well as the visits of distinguished personages, have largely contributed to render Ischl more attractive in the eyes of other visitors. An Alpine village in its primitive condition is neither clean nor pleasing to the eye. The Ischl of the days when Dr. Wirer first settled in it must have been a much less attractive place than that which now exists. At one time, indeed, cretins and cripples abounded. The general health of the population has improved in proportion as the sanitary conditions under which the people live have become more perfect. Nature has been aided by art to render the spot most enjoyable. Thackeray wrote that a good test of the impression produced by the great writers of Queen Anne's reign was whether we feel that we should like to associate with them on terms of intimacy, and he pronounced Swift to be one who would not stand such a test. I think an equally good test of the attractiveness of a health resort to be whether those who have spent several days in it would like to return. Now I feel sure that others who have sojourned at Ischl will agree with me in affirming that it is pre-eminently a place to be revisited.

CHAPTER IX.

GASTEIN.

HAD the "Carlsbad Resolutions," embodying the policy of Metternich, and forming the basis of the ill-omened Holy Alliance of Continental Sovereigns against the wishes and aspirations of their people for constitutional freedom, been alone associated with the principal Bohemian watering-place, it would long be noteworthy in the history of this century. Whilst vying with Carlsbad as a health resort for invalids throughout the world, Gastein is conspicuous in the annals of Europe owing to the momentous Convention concluded here between Count Bismarck von Schönhausen and Count Blome, on the 14th of August, 1865, and signed at Salzburg six days later by the King of Prussia and the Emperor of Austria. The Gastein Convention was Count Bismarck's most daring and skilful diplomatic feat. Its conclusion was regarded as ending the Schleswig-Holstein dispute, whereas the Convention led, as may have been designed and foreseen by the astute Prussian Minister, to the great object of his life, the permanent exclusion of Austria from Germany, a severance which was followed by the Franco-German war, by the elevation of the King of Prussia to the dignity of German Emperor, and by the union of Germany under the headship of Prussia. In any case, then, Gastein has been consecrated, to use Goethe's word, by the presence of illustrious and potent personages. No visitor can easily forget this, whether he goes there out of curiosity or in order to be rejuvenated by its waters. The map of Europe has been re-modelled here during the leisure hours of elderly men who came to bathe and feel young again.

Whilst Gastein is a place much frequented by those who have exercised no small influence upon mankind, it has an interest of its own, apart from the mineral springs for which it is famous, and it has also a long and eventful history. I shall content myself with a simple reference to the legend which attributes the discovery of the hot mineral springs at Gastein to a wounded stag being found in the year 680 engaged in a species of self-cure, or rather self-help, and that tells how certain Christians fled here from Rome to escape persecution in the reign of Tiberius.

The facts are quite as curious as any legend, and they have the advantage of being authentic.

Many centuries ago the valley of Gastein was as famous for yielding the precious metals as California and Australia have been in our day. The aborigines, who were of Celtic origin, carried on mining here before they were subdued by the Romans, and this locality was included in the Roman province of Noricum, an event which occurred in the year 15 B.C. Mining was prosecuted with great vigour by the Romans, who employed slaves to work in the mines, just as the Russians now employ convicts. After a time mining ceased, and it was not resumed till 790, when, as is stated in an extant record, the mines, which had been worked by the Romans and abandoned for many years, were again reopened. When the Archbishopric of Salzburg was founded in the ninth century, a part of the district embracing these mines was attached to it, and the produce of the mines formed a large portion of the Archbishop's income. In a document dated 890, in which the boundaries of this district are described, the name "Gastuna" appears for the first time. Yet it was not till the fourteenth century that the entire Gastein valley passed under the temporal power of the Archbishops of Salzburg. At the beginning of the fifteenth century, people from all parts of Europe flocked to this valley, and some made fortunes by gold-mining and more by lending money and buying the gold product.

When the mining industry was in full vigour, the preaching of Luther agitated men's minds, and his doctrines found many adherents amongst the miners and capitalists of Gastein. The Archbishop of Salzburg was professionally adverse to the spread of the new doctrines; but the heretics were allowed to mine the precious metals in comparative peace till 1588, when a decree went forth from Salzburg that all non-Catholics were to quit the Gastein valley. The result was to diminish the number of workers so greatly that the returns from the mines were largley diminished. In 1591, Archbishop Wolfgang Dietrich, who had issued the edict, visited the valley, and became convinced that if it were rigorously enforced, he would be the loser in pocket. Accordingly, he assured the miners who had remained that they would be undisturbed in their religious profession if they continued their labours. Even had not religious intolerance seriously interfered with the prosperity of the valley, its brightest days were over. Prices had gone up for articles of consumption; the value of the precious metals had fallen consequent upon the opening up of the New World. Moreover, the discovery of the way to India round the Cape of Good Hope proved disastrous not only to the commerce of Venice and of other Italian cities, but also to this remote valley, and, while mining was steadily growing less profitable, the Archbishops of Salzburg became more vehement in their determination to drive away the Protestant miners. Five hundred Protestants were forced into exile in the years 1614 and 1615. Between those years and 1631, as many as 330 were banished. In 1713, the last and largest exodus took place, when 700 persons went to find new homes in America and East Prussia, where they might work in quietness and worship God undisturbed. The capitalists followed the workers, and the industry of mining in the valley of Gastein dwindled into insignificance. Many mines which were then closed have never been reopened. Fifty miners are now at work. The annual yield of silver has been valued at £400, and of gold at £3,500.

The effect of the edicts of the Archbishops of Salzburg was to depopulate the valley of Gastein, and to cause an amount of actual suffering and loss for which there was no valid excuse, and for which no compensation could be given. Several Protestants lived in Salzburg, and they were suffered to remain undisturbed. But an indirect punishment was inflicted upon them also. At that time the mineral waters of Gastein were becoming as celebrated as its mines, and their healing properties attracted many sufferers. The Archbishop forbade the Protestants of Salzburg to visit Gastein in order to be cured of their ailments. It is now long since the Archbishops of Salzburg exercised temporal as well as spiritual authority over the Gasteiners. If the most energetic scourge of heretics amongst them could revisit the earth, he would be satisfied with the religious condition of the dwellers in the valley, which contains 3972 inhabitants, of whom two only are Protestants.

Centuries elapsed after the discovery of the mineral springs at Gastein before they were generally used and appreciated. It is probable that the inhabitants bathed in the mineral water simply because it was hot. The unlettered savage who can get a warm bath without trouble is quite ready to take it. In 1436, the first known patient went to Gastein to be cured; this was the Duke Frederick who was afterwards Emperor. That the reputation of the waters rapidly increased is shown by the fact that a hospital was established at Gastein in 1489. Though I shall use the name Gastein, as that which is most familiar, I may state once for all that the full and correct name is Wildbad-Gastein.

One of the first persons pretending to a knowledge of physic who visited the place and analysed the mineral water was Theophrastus Bombastus Paracelsus, his visit taking place after the first hotel, occupying the site of the present Straubinger's Hotel, was erected, in 1590. Dr. Duelli was the earliest doctor who resided at Gastein during the season in order to direct patients how to use the waters, and it was in 1671 that his practice in this capacity began. The Badeschloss Hotel, where the German Emperor William the First stayed during his last visit, was built by the Archbishop of Salzburg in 1794 for the accommodation of princes and potentates, and not till 1807 were persons of less distinction permitted to take up their quarters in it. During many years of its existence as a health resort, the building of a new house has been the chief event in Gastein's history. The open space there is very limited, and the accommodation for visitors is so restricted still that it is impossible to find a vacant room in the height of the season. Till the year 1875 it was the rule to travel by coach from Salzburg, a tedious and wearisome journey; but in that year the railway passed Lend, and now visitors can drive to Gastein from the Lend Station in four hours.

I have three German books before me describing Gastein and its baths. The first, dated 1881, is the third edition of Dr. Pröll's elaborate work, the author having practised as a physician at Gastein for a generation, and taken hundreds of baths himself, as well as prescribed them to his patients; the second, dated 1885, is the fourth edition of the work of Dr. Bunzel, another physician who has long practised there; and the third, dated 1885, is entitled "A Medical, Historical, and Topographical Sketch of Gastein," by Dr. von Härdtl and three others filling official positions in that watering-place. In none of these works, nor in others treating of Gastein which I have consulted, is reference made to a visitor who is quite as important a personage as any Sovereign whose name is associated with it. This is William von Humboldt. In his "Letters to Charlotte," a book by which Humboldt is better known than by his works on philosophy and philology, and by which he will be longer and more favourably remembered than by his services as a Prussian ambassador and statesman, a most interesting account is given of Gastein when he visited it in 1827 for the first time. Since he saw it then the material changes in the place are few, whilst the journey to it from Lend by road is similar to that which he describes; the road is somewhat improved, and that is all. The visitor still sees, as Humboldt saw, the River Ache dash down for the last time in its headlong career from the source to the Salzach, near Lend. Still, as in his day, must the carriage be drawn by many horses at a snail's pace up the precipitous road which winds through the Klamm Pass. After a long and toilsome ascent the Gastein valley is reached, and it looks the more beautiful in contrast to the gloomy passage through the rocks which has been traversed. The broad green winding valley is dotted with houses. Dorf-Gastein is the first village; next comes Hof-Gastein, whither mineral water is conveyed from the higher ground. The Emperor Francis the First gave permission for this to be done. Out of gratitude, the inhabitants have erected a bronze bust of their benefactor. In this village there is a military hospital. Some persons who do not like the noise of the resounding waterfall at Gastein prefer to stay in Hof-Gastein for treatment. Beyond this village the ascent becomes steep again, and after an hour and a half's drive one's journey's end is reached. The valley, which is about thirty miles in length, extends far above Gastein till the foot of the mountains is attained, whence the water which forms and feeds the River Ache rushes down from the glaciers far above.

Every visitor to Gastein, since it has been a place of resort for the ailing, is most impressed with the waterfall and most affected by the air. Gastein lies at an elevation of about 3000 feet above the sea, and the air has that pure Alpine character which is both invigorating and enlivening. One feels lighter, so to speak, after breathing it. Some invalids are benefited by it as much as by drinking or bathing in the mineral waters. They eat with greater appetite; they walk without being so soon fatigued; they enjoy in mature age that sweet and refreshing sleep which is the chief blessing of childhood. Yet, whether this happy result be experienced or not, there is no question about the impression which the waterfall makes upon them. Though not the largest, the waterfall at Gastein is the longest, and, perhaps, the noisiest in Europe. It loses none of its force in the hottest weather. On the contrary, the volume of water is greater in the height of summer than at any other season of the year, for then it is that the sun melts the snow on the high mountain tops and the River Ache is swollen to its utmost bounds. The aspect of the fall is striking, but it is nothing in comparison with that of Niagara. Nevertheless the noise at Gastein seems greater than at Niagara, or rather the ear is more affected by it. The difference between the two is equivalent to that between the baying of a bloodhound and the barking of a pug. The pug makes more noise; the bloodhound emits more sound. If the water fell sheer down at Gastein as at Niagara, the effect would be far more imposing, the descent being upwards of 600 feet. As it is, the water rushes down a slope instead of leaping from a height, its course is broken by rocks, and though the noise is increased by this the grandeur of the spectacle is lessened.

In the day when William von Humboldt visited Gastein, as in our own, the waterfall has been a subject of concern, as well as an object to be admired. Then the nervous patients who came to Gastein for relief could not sit in comfort or sleep at all within sound of the rushing water. It was impossible to converse in comfort in a room near the fall. This is equally true now. Humboldt notes that he did not dislike the noise, though he found it disagreeable to strain his voice in conversation. In our day nervous patients suffer as they did in his, and the waterfall is regarded by many visitors with repulsion and horror. Humboldt mentions that such persons take long walks in order to get away from the noise. It is not uncommon for those who are sensitive to sounds to live lower down in the valley. As for Humboldt, he was never weary of gazing upon the waterfall, and he was never disturbed by its din. He notes that he took a bath at four o'clock in the morning, stayed an hour in the water, and went back to bed, where he slept for two hours.

It was remarked as something extraordinary that the Empress of Austria when she was here recently should take a bath so early as four o'clock, as the hour for opening the baths is five, and most persons bathe between six and seven. In one respect the "cure" was pursued half a century ago in the same fashion as at present. When Humboldt was at Gastein, few persons drank the waters; few drink them now. Some doctors prescribe them, and Dr. Pröll considers their internal use to be quite as curative as their external application. He remarks, with perfect justice, that for centuries after the waters of Carlsbad were known to effect cures no one thought of drinking them, whereas now there is far more drinking than bathing at Carlsbad, whilst the results from their internal use are even more striking than those from taking baths alone. In like manner the Gastein waters may yet enjoy a renown hereafter greater than they have now, should the fashion of drinking them become general. Though Gastein has grown since Humboldt's visits, a complaint which visitors made in his day is made still: it is that the walks on level ground are very few and short. Many patients being weak and elderly, the necessity of ascending a hill with the view of taking a long walk is a serious drawback to enjoyment, and may even retard the cure in several cases. Humboldt paid his first visit in 1827, and his last in 1830. In a letter written in 1830, he states that the baths improved his appetite, and he laments that the food is bad. Being so hungry, however, he was able to eat food from which he would turn with repulsion elsewhere. Some visitors still grumble about the food. For my own part I had no reason to complain. When one considers the distance from which everything has to be brought, and the difficulties of transport, one is inclined to wonder that the living is so good. In these circumstances it is a matter of course that prices should be high.

Life at Gastein is very earnest. People visit it to be cured, and not for pleasure. A band plays twice a day, but no other amusement is provided for the visitors. Patients go to bed and get up early; they eat little during the day, and they remain as much out of doors as possible. Above all things they must regularly consult a physician, and strictly follow his advice. To take a bath without seeing a doctor is held to be tempting Providence and incurring the risk of sudden death. As Dr. Pröll puts it, such conduct is as foolish as that of the person who should go to a chemist's shop, procure a dose of strong medicine, swallow it, and then have recourse to a doctor for advice.

The most remarkable thing connected with the waters of Gastein is that, whilst powerful in their action, they are very poor in mineral ingredients. Chemists style them "indifferent" waters; the word is misleading if taken in its ordinary signification, but what is meant is that they have little chemical importance. Such waters, of which many exist, are classed as "acratothermæ," the word being a compound, meaning unmixed or pure [mineral] waters. Mistakes have arisen from confounding ἄκρατος, unmixed, with ἀκρατής, weak, and concluding that waters so designated were powerless. It is easier, however, to settle the meaning of words than to explain why the waters which contain so little mineral substance should prove curative. The chief ingredient is silicilic acid, but what the effects of that acid are on the skin or on the inner organs of the body is a mystery. Of late years it is the fashion to solve problems by the aid of electricity. In default of any other explanation of its action, Gastein water is said to exercise a powerful action upon the human system because there is so much electricity in it. The conductivity of the water as compared with distilled water is said to be as six to one. Both Dr. Pröll and Dr. Bunzel insist upon the electrical character of the water, though the former confesses that he is sceptical as to the electric shocks which some patients report to have occurred while bathing, and he attributes this to excessive sensitiveness coupled with a vivid imagination on their parts. But Dr. von Härdtl and others entirely differ from their colleagues, maintaining that the talk about electricity is perfectly idle, and stating that, according to experiments made at Munich with

Gastein and Iser water, each displayed the same electrical conductivity without being identical in healing power. So long as medical authorities of equal note display that happy divergence of view which leads to so many experiments and so much discussion, the public must take the side which pleases it the best, and at present the action of Gastein water is generally though, as I believe, erroneously supposed to have some connexion with electricity.

That the water of Gastein is hot when it issues from the earth is the one fact which cannot be denied. A hot water bath has a certain specific action, whether the water be plain or mineralised. If hot mineral water at Gastein acts better or differently than hot baths wherein plain water is the sole agent, then Gastein hot mineral water has a marked superiority over hot plain water. It is one thing, however, to note that mineral water acts in a particular way, and it is something quite different and far more difficult to explain the cause or the manner of its action. Professor Seegen, after many years' practice at Carlsbad, found that the Carlsbad waters produced an alleviation of the worst symptoms in cases of diabetes such as could not be induced by any other water or medicine; he candidly admitted, however, his inability to explain how the result was obtained. Writers about mineral waters would do well to display a modesty such as his, which was that of a man of great talent and varied scientific attainments. That Gastein mineral water is curative may be accepted as a fact; but the reasons are as obscure now as they were when the legendary stag resorted to it for relief in the year 680.

Having drunk Gastein mineral water, I found that it did not differ in taste from ordinary warm water. I bathed in it several times without any appreciable result. Others have been less fortunate. I have collected particulars concerning many persons who have suffered for drinking and bathing in the water without medical advice. Dr. Pröll narrates how a man came to Gastein in July, 1860, suffering from an affection of the spine; how he took a bath shortly after his arrival, and felt so much the worse that he started off the following day, under the impression that the mineral waters were injurious. He cites the case of a lady who climbed a hill after her first bath, felt faint, fell, and broke her arm; but he omits to say that climbing a hill after a hot bath is a mistake, whether the water be mineralised or not. The best example advanced by Dr. Pröll is that drawn from his personal experience. He took too many baths, and he felt the worse for doing so. He fails to see that no stronger reason needs be assigned in support of his contention that every patient should consult a doctor before bathing. As a patient, he required advice as much as, if not more than, any layman. So long as a physician cannot cure himself, so long must the word "impossible" remain in the dictionaries, despite Bonaparte's objection to it.

Two things seem to demonstrate the potency of Gastein mineral water, and one of them shows that the mountain air of the locality cannot alone effect the cures which are wrought. First, the patients in the public hospital are for the most part mountaineers; they are born and bred in the neighbourhood; they are ailing when they begin the treatment, and they are cured by bathing in and drinking the water: second, withered flowers placed in the water revive and regain their lost perfume. I tried an experiment with flowers, and it succeeded perfectly. I divided the flowers into two bunches, placing one bunch in a tumblerful of ordinary water and the other in Gastein mineral water. After the lapse of a few hours the wild flowers, which had been plucked the day before and were to all appearance quite dead, revived and remained fresh for several days, whilst those in the plain water remained withered and scentless. It is said that Gastein is emphatically a bath for old men, a place in which they renew their youth. If the water acts upon them as it does upon the flowers, they ought not only to grow young again, but become evergreens. The flowers are affected in the course of a few hours, but some patients are less sensitive to the action of the water. Dr. Pröll mentions the case of a patient who felt no good result till eleven months after he had quitted Gastein. This would imply that, in certain cases, the "cure" lasts one month, and that the rest of the year must pass away before the patient gets well enough to be ready to resume the "cure." Such a "cure" may eventually be radical, but it cannot be called rapid.

For those who are not debilitated or incapacitated from walking at all, there are many pleasant excursions to be made in the neighbourhood of Gastein. An hour's walk up the valley brings one to Böckstein, which is more charmingly situated than Gastein, but where there are no mineral springs. On the other hand, the drinking water at Böckstein is delicious, being very cold and very pure. A hydropathic establishment attracts many persons to Böckstein. Still farther up the valley the scenery is most striking. In other valleys, not far distant, as fine views can be had, while several lakes are most picturesquely situated. Among them the Pokhart is by far the largest and the most curious. Its water is impregnated with arsenic; no living thing exists in or near it; the colour of the water is a deep black; in fact, the Pokhart lake resembles the Dead Sea.

Notwithstanding the limited space near the springs

at Gastein, there are several walks adjoining them which are both well planned and well kept. At short intervals there are seats for the weary and shelters from the heat or rain. Perhaps it is because the visitors have idle hands that the seats and resting places are covered with written inscriptions. Germans often indulge in verses praising Gastein. Americans inscribe their names, their addresses, and the dates of their visit. No one, it may be said, is benefited by these inscriptions, and I think that visitors would act more rationally if they refrained from leaving these traces of their sojourn. Yet there is a great deal of human nature in these inscriptions. If the pre-historic dwellers in caves had not made their marks on pieces of bone, some of the most curious tracings in the Christy collection of the remains of the cave men would not have survived to excite and gratify our curiosity.

The late Dr. Hill Burton, in the chapter in his "History of Scotland" treating of archæology, gives some explanations respecting the old inscriptions which appear as sensible as they are ingenious. Historians have puzzled themselves to extract a meaning from these runes. Sometimes the meaning seems clear, and sometimes the whole becomes vague. Dr. Burton surmised that some people of ancient Britain, like idlers in general, might have made their marks on stone to pass the time, and might have impressed on the stones nothing more weighty than their names, their places of abode, or their passing fancies. At intervals a real story may have formed the substance of a rune, and the puzzle would be the greater to separate the idle memorandum from the record of some interesting fact. I was the more struck with this on observing in a secluded spot near the waterfall at Gastein a few lines of doggerel verse which would furnish materials for a story to a novelist in want of a subject. The lines are few, so I may quote them; the story itself requires little elucidation. At the beginning is the sketch of a young lady's head, and then follow these lines, "To Helen":

> Riches, source of so much woe,
> How happy would you be,
> If in a cottage you would dwell,
> With none to love but me.

Immediately after, in a lady's hand and with a lady's punctuation, are these words: "Helen is much obliged; thanks for the offer but has already accepted number one. Hopes to see you in Paris." It scarcely needs to be pointed out that Helen's wooer did not deserve to succeed. He appeals to Helen to be happy with him, not to make him happy. This is not the way in which to touch a woman's heart. As Coleridge wrote, with his usual penetration: " A man's desire is for the woman, but a woman's desire is for the desire of the man." Helen was quite right in preferring number one to the suitor who was unable to touch her heart.

In describing the approach to Gastein I mentioned that the valley which used to be populated with Protestants now contains but two only. Many of the visitors to Gastein are Protestants, and a German Protestant Church has been built for their use, and it is secured against interference by being vested in the German Emperor. I should not omit to state that Gastein mineral water, besides rejuvenating the aged, has the further virtues of rendering ladies' faces more beautiful, of healing wounds, and stopping seasickness. Dr. Pröll is my authority for these statements. If all that he and others write in praise of this water be literally true, then it can work more miracles than the water of Lourdes.

The mere sightseer is not wanted at Gastein. Most of the fifty houses composing the place are provided with baths, and every visitor is expected to use the baths or drink the mineral water. Complaints are made by the resident physicians that patients are sent to them who are incurable or who require surgical treatment. Indeed, it is common to say, when all other baths and remedies fail, "Try Gastein."

I have used Dr. Pröll's German work on Gastein when making extracts, and I may now turn to one by him in English, entitled "Gastein: Its Springs and Climate," and quote a few passages. A list of twenty forms of disease is given, each of which might be benefited by treatment here. At the close of the list, Dr. Pröll lays down the following "General Rule.—All patients who are submissive, and suffering for a long time from any disease—even when its seat be unknown—which is ameliorated by a moderate amount of food, and are without fever, may be sent to the baths of Gastein with hope of success." He is strongly of opinion that no one should visit Gastein who has a natural disposition to oppose and disobey the physician.

Dr. Pröll supplies information as to the best season for taking the "cure" on the spot. Out of the detailed reasons given by him for the choice of a particular month, I select the more noteworthy. He pronounces the period from the 1st of May to the 15th of June as the best for those "who require the special care of a physician, and who expect to find in him a counsellor and friend, and those who require special nursing and care from the attendants." The period from the 15th of June to the 15th of August is suitable for those "who need warmth for travelling and for the sojourn; who could order their rooms five months in advance, or who are not particular in the choice of a room; who do not need special care from the physician or attendants, and who have only the autumn for the repose necessary after the baths."

Between the 15th of August and the 15th of October is the time for those "who need preparatory treatment during two or three months at other springs before coming to Gastein; who need constant fine weather and warmer than in spring . . . and those who suffer from biliousness, piles, and a tendency to anger and apoplexy should especially select this season."

Though Gastein is not an inviting place in winter, yet, according to Dr. Pröll, there are many who may visit it for treatment between the 15th of October and the 30th of April. He says that amongst them are the persons who cannot come at any other season and who have no liberty of choice; he also says that "the winter is favourable for those who fear the temptation of mountain-climbing; or who suffer from any loathsome or contagious disease." His conclusion is that "winter, spring, and autumn are the most favourable seasons for the cure; the best time is from the 15th of August to the 15th of October. The least favourable is the summer, and it should be chosen only by the rich and by those not seriously ill."

Since the German Emperor, William the First, and Prince Bismarck visited Gastein, patriotic Prussians have followed their example in the hope of being benefited also. When William von Humboldt was here, few North Germans were undergoing treatment. Now, the harsher accents of the North are heard as often in the hotels and streets as the softer tones of South German or Austrian speech. The French eschew Gastein, and the English visitors are few in number. In the *Gastein Chronicle*, which has been kept since 1680, and wherein every visitor may make an entry, it is recorded that three Englishmen were here in 1800, and that they were the first persons of their nation who had visited Gastein. Yet no person from any part of Austria, except the Emperor and the Empress, or from any foreign country, has attracted so much notice or made a greater mark here than Prince Bismarck. The Gasteiners are wont to boast, *Gastuna tantum una*. Indeed, there is but one Gastein, and Prince Bismarck is its hero.

CHAPTER X.

MERAN.

"Go to Meran and eat grapes," is the advice given to many patients at Carlsbad, Marienbad, Kissingen, and Tarasp. Others, who have bathed in or drunk the mineral waters at these places, are ordered to go to Meran by their physicians with a view to enjoy an "after-cure" in change of air and scene. Many sufferers, to whom mineral waters bring no relief, visit Meran for the sake of its climate, more especially in winter. In the autumn it is largely frequented by tourists, who are attracted by its beauties. Few spots in Tyrol are more charming than Meran, nor does any one present such varied points of interest. The invalid with a delicate chest and the sightseer with an insatiable curiosity, the student of history and the student of science, can all find at Meran something to benefit or interest them.

Though Meran has lost the importance it possessed

while the capital of Tyrol, it is no longer the dwindling place which it was for years. Since the opening, in 1871, of the branch line of railway between it and Botzen, the number of visitors has multiplied, and new houses and hotels have been erected to accommodate them. As many as thirty villas have been built during the year that is past. The drawback now seems to be the too rapid growth of the place. A health resort loses many attractions as it increases in size. The drainage almost invariably deteriorates as house is added to house. Thus the loveliest spot may be ruined by over-popularity. In some notices of Meran the season is said to begin in October and end in April. This is not quite accurate. According to Dr. Pircher, one of the resident physicians, the season lasts the whole year round; in other words, there are classes of ailments for which a sojourn here is desirable in spring, summer, autumn, and winter. For the largest number of invalids, however, it is a place of resort during the winter months. The climate is the cheapest and most certain "cure" in Meran.

The grape cure season begins in September and continues to the end of October. It has been practised at Meran for fifty years. Like other novelties in medical treatment, this form of cure was once as absurdly over-rated and misapplied as hydropathy till persons who had been quite as fanatical as Priestnitz were compelled by experience to admit that drinking cold water and wrapping one's self in wet sheets might not be a sovereign remedy for every malady. When writing about Baden and Vöslau, I mentioned how the grape cure was pursued at both places. At Meran, however, the cure is conducted in a still more serious fashion. The grapes themselves are better adapted for the purpose than any which are to be found elsewhere. They resemble English hothouse grapes more than those grown on the Continent in the open air. They are very pulpy and luscious. They are carefully picked, and they are cheap, the average price per pound being threepence.

Two physicians practising at Meran, Dr. Kuhn and Dr. Pircher, have written about the grape cure as pursued there. They are both men of note and experience in their profession, and they differ in opinion on an important point. Dr. Kuhn states that the grape stones are not to be swallowed on any account, and he adds that if swallowed they are certain to upset the digestion. Dr. Pircher, on the other hand, intimates that swallowing the grape stones does good instead of harm by facilitating the digestive processes. Some other doctors, I believe, tell their patients to please themselves in this matter. Another disputed point is whether the expressed juice of the grapes may not be taken with advantage. Dr. Pircher replies with an emphatic negative, threatening those who swallow the juice with colic as a penalty. Dr. Kuhn is quite as emphatic in recommending those persons to take the juice whose mouths have been irritated by continuously eating grapes.

As regards the cure itself, it is not so pleasant as it sounds, and I write this after an experimental trial extending over several days. All the doctors agree that no effect will be produced unless two pounds of grapes are eaten daily. The maximum dose is nine pounds. I managed to eat about five pounds daily, and thought that I had done enough for an experiment. I was quite satisfied in one respect. I should imagine breaking stones at the roadside to be a somewhat monotonous as well as exhausting employment, yet I can well suppose that a moment arrives to a patient under the grape cure when such a form of toil seems preferable to that of eating grapes all day. But the patient is not always relieved from toil when the day ends. He is haunted with grapes in his sleep, and dreams of having to eat a double dose or die.

The first thing the grape eater finds is that his appetite is not increased. He may have been told that he will feel hungrier the more grapes he eats, but his experience will probably be similar to that of an American boy with oysters. This boy had been told that eating oysters gave one an appetite for dinner. He complained that after eating half-a-bushel he did not feel so hungry as when he began. The swallowing of from two to eight pounds weight of grapes induces a sensation of complete satiety. Our eighteenth century writers were fond of depicting how soon and sadly all pleasures cloyed when indulged to excess. If they could revisit Meran during the grape cure season, they would find plenty of subjects wherewith to point such morals. But it may be supposed that living entirely upon grapes has many compensations. Vegetarians are fond of asserting that their heads are so clear and light, and that they have pleasures in life unknown to the eater of meat; moreover, they are very fond of eating eggs and cheese, and of drinking milk, things which cannot, I think, be classed as vegetables by any one except a very light-headed vegetarian. Grapes may fairly be called light as a diet; yet the effect of eating them is heavy. If vegetables produce as many unpleasant sensations, which I should consider most probable, then the meat eater is to be envied both by the eater of the fruit or vegetables. He is generally unconscious of the sufferings from flatulence which frequently follow a vegetable diet, and his mouth is not irritated as is that of the eater of grapes.

I have styled the grape cure a serious one; I must add that it requires the exercise of much patience in those who follow it. Dr. Pircher is minute in his directions to patients; they are not doing their duty if they merely swallow grapes in a rapid and unmethodical manner. He tells them to be careful that the bunches are freshly cut, and also that "they must take each grape separately, examine it carefully in order to ascertain that it is quite ripe and that it does not contain any insect, the presence of an insect being indicated by a perforation of the skin. When the grape is placed in the mouth it must not be bitten, as is generally done, but it must be gently pressed by the tongue against the hard gums and sucked so as to draw out the juice; the grape skin must be spat out." He goes on to add, as I have mentioned already, that the stones are to be swallowed, and he continues by giving a warning against squeezing the skins between the teeth. In this case, as in many others, Dr. Pircher displays that fondness for detail which is characteristic of some medical writers in German, who consider themselves to be much more profound than their English brethren. No English medical man would think of telling a patient how to eat grapes, any more than he would think of telling them, as Dr. Halwaceck does in his work on Carlsbad, that it is wise to carry an umbrella when rain threatens. An English medical man does not assume that he is addressing children when writing a guide to a watering-place. A German is at once more paternal and prosy. After quoting what Dr. Pircher has written, I should not omit to add a calculation which I made. If grapes are eaten as he directs, the average rate of consumption will be one a minute. In a pound of the grapes supplied at Meran there are about 300. Now the patient begins with one kilogramme, which is upwards of two pounds, and he takes an additional pound daily till the maximum dose of nine pounds is reached. On the first day the task is comparatively simple. After ten hours' steady exertion, the two pounds can be disposed of in strict obedience with the doctor's precise orders. But, by the time the dose reaches five pounds, the problem occurs as to how to eat the grapes at the rate of one a minute in the course of a day of twenty-four hours, seeing that twenty-four hours will have elapsed before the whole are consumed. When the dose reaches eight pounds, sixty hours will be required to take it in due form. Dr. Johnson said of Shakespeare that "panting Time toils after him in vain." At Meran the grape-eating patient must pant after Time, and do so in despair. I may hazard the conjecture, by way of helping to solve the problem, that the patients at Meran eat grapes quicker and less systematically than they are enjoined to do in the pages of Dr. Pircher's work.

Before describing the attractions of Meran as a

winter residence, I shall briefly mention the other forms of "cure" in vogue there. Amongst them the milk and whey cures are pre-eminent. Meran cows' milk is remarkable for its excellence; the whey made from goats' milk in Meran is exceedingly rich in sugar. The patient who is under a milk diet gets milk alone; but he gets plenty of it, the dose being nearly a quart every three hours. If, after existing on milk for a week, the patient longs for something more substantial, he is allowed a roll or two soaked in milk; at the end of a fortnight he is given a little meat, and after three weeks' treatment he is either quite recovered or he ought to be, the fault being his own if the cure is not complete. Milk is obtainable at different times in the year; the period of the whey cure, however, begins in April and ends with May. Whey is drunk in the morning, and some mineral water is often taken along with it. Those persons whose cases are not adapted for the milk or whey cure may find benefit from koumiss, prepared from cows' milk. The dose at the beginning of the treatment is an imperial quart taken in two portions daily—the one in the morning, the other in the afternoon. The quantity taken is gradually increased till the daily dose is three imperial quarts.

All the foregoing forms of "cure" are not peculiar to Meran, though they are pursued there in a more systematic fashion than in other places. The last I have to mention cannot be had in like perfection elsewhere. It is a plant-juice cure, and is available in the spring only, when certain plants unfold their first green leaves on the slopes of the Alps. The juice is expressed from them and the patient drinks it. It may interest the botanist to learn the names of the plants so employed; they are *Achillæa millefolium, Nasturtium aquaticum, Rumex acetosa, Ruta graviolens, Leontodon taraxacum, Urtica dioica,* and *Menyanthes trifoliata.* The decoction is green in colour and bitter in taste. Cases of indigestion and poverty of blood are said to be benefited by this "cure," which is practised from the middle of March till the middle of April.

Yet the chief, the most effective, and by far the pleasantest "cure" at Meran is the climate, and especially the climate in winter. Tourists visit it in summer; invalids spend the winter here. Meran lies at an elevation of 1000 feet towards the upper end of one of the widest valleys in Central Europe. It is built on the River Passer, which falls into the Adige. The valley is open towards the south; on the other sides a girdle of granitic and porphyritic mountains rises to a height of from 6000 feet to 10,000 feet. These mountains protect it from the winds which blow at higher points; when the storms rage and the rain falls round their mountain summits, not a breath of air causes the leaves to rustle on the trees in Meran. Rain seldom falls in the valley, even when it is pouring on the higher slopes of the mountains. The finest weather is during the autumn and winter months. A series of observations extending over ten years shows that the yearly average of perfectly clear days—that is, days when the sky is cloudless and the sun bright—is 127, and these are apportioned as follows: 48 in the months of December, January, and February, 25 in the spring months, 21 in the summer, and 33 in the autumn. It is rarely that the sun does not shine brightly during a few hours of every winter's day. There is least wind during the coldest months, and most rain during the hottest. A cloudless sky, warm sunshine, a dry and still air, and an equable temperature, are the characteristics of a Meran winter. The health of the inhabitants testifies in favour of the climate. At several places where consumptive invalids are sent to be relieved or cured, the mortality from consumption is very large among the inhabitants. Not so in Meran. While in Vienna 66 in every 1000 are afflicted with disease of the lungs, in Meran the number is 12. The death-rate is very low. Out of a population of 5236 the average death-rate during ten years was at the rate of 23 annually, of whom a third attained the age of 60, and 5 per cent. of all who died were upwards of 80. Shrubs and trees which do not grow where the climate is ungenial flourish in the gardens of Meran; among them are the aloe, the oleander, and the magnolia.

Nothing that had been written about Meran as a winter place of abode produced so much effect as the fact of the Empress of Austria staying there during the winter of 1870-71, and repeating her visit the following winter. It is true that the opening of railway communication, first by the completion of the Brenner railway from Innsbruck to Botzen in 1866, and second by that of the branch line between Botzen and Meran in 1871, had prepared the way for visitors; yet the sojourn of the Empress was the best possible advertisement, making many persons curious to know about a place which would not otherwise have attracted their notice. The increase in the number of those spending the winter in Meran has been very large during the last ten years. In 1854, when Dr. Pircher first began to practise there, the number of invalids who had selected it for their winter home was 60; fifteen years later the number had risen to upwards of 1000; it is now upwards of 3000. Yet there is a real winter at Meran, though it is mild and healthy. Those who would escape winter altogether must follow the swallows to Egypt or Madeira, Sicily or Africa. While those who praise the climate of Meran admit that it is not so warm as that of the Riviera, they also contend that it suits many delicate persons far better, inasmuch as it is more equable, and chiefly because there is less disturbance from wind. The difference between sunshine and shade is much greater along the Riviera, and the cold days are more trying. When the sun does not shine at Cannes or Nice, Mentone or San Remo, the invalids suffer dreadfully, and it is no unusual occurrence for the sky to be completely clouded for days together. There the cold is felt indoors even more than in the open air; many rooms are without fireplaces, and the invalids shiver, pine, and die. At Meran, on the contrary, the houses are comfortably warmed, and, though the thermometer may fall very low during the night, the invalid does not feel cold. I am assured by those who have wintered in Italy and Meran that they prefer the latter. I have seen enough of it to be convinced that the stillness of the air is marvellous. When the sun shines brightly and there is no wind, cold is but slightly felt, provided the air be dry. I have walked about without an overcoat in Manitoba—where the air is marvellously dry—when the thermometer was below zero, and I did not feel so cold as I have done in London with an overcoat when it was forty degrees higher. The air is very dry in Meran.

Professor C. W. C. Fuchs, in the interesting "Studies" concerning the geology, climate, and plant-life around Meran, which he recently published, gives the result of his personal experience when wintering there and at Nice. He likens the Nice winter to early spring in Central Germany. At Meran the nights are wintry, and the days are those of early summer elsewhere. In sheltered spots the ice does not melt, and the sight is not uncommon of persons skating in their shirt-sleeves. What occurs at Meran in winter resembles what occurs in the higher Alpine regions during summer, where the sun streams from a blue sky by day, and where the nights have a frosty look and feeling, yet where in sheltered spots the violet blows and strawberries ripen. The Meran winter is the hot summer on the snow-line of the Alps transferred to the wide and windless valley of the Adige.

The valley is fertile and thickly populated. Growing grapes and fruit, and rearing cattle, are the occupations of the people. Meran fruit has a wide reputation, and it is despatched in large quantities not only to all parts of Austria and Germany, but even as far as Russia. Though the grapes are so good, the wine made from them is poor, the peasants giving too little attention to the process of wine-making. These peasants are laborious and well-to-do. Their farms are freeholds, and primogeniture is the rule. Most farms have been in the same family for generations. The eldest son lives on and by his farm; the younger sons either work under him or live upon strangers. The people are pious; they are very fond of outward shows and ceremonies, and the men religiously observe the feast days, of which there are about two a week. On these days the women work harder than usual, while the men occupy themselves with playing cards and drinking wine. Very large quantities of wine are consumed by the peasants. Dr. Pircher is my authority for saying that many peasants who never drink a drop of water, and drink far too much wine, live to a good old age. They eat heartily and heavily; five meals a day are required to appease their appetites; at each meal smoked meat, maize, and black bread are eaten. The bread is baked four times a year, so it is generally stale and satisfying. In speech the people are Germans, and they show no trace of the Italian blood and characteristics which are conspicuous in other parts of South Tyrol. It is probable, however, that the stock is very mixed, as the people of many nations have successively occupied this part of Europe.

In the work by Professor Fuchs, already referred to, it is shown that no other part of the Alpine region is richer in lessons for the geologist than this one. Its physical history is depicted on the rocks. There was a time when this broad, lovely, and fertile valley was filled with a glacier several thousand feet thick, and when the peaks of the highest mountains, covered with snow, were the only prominent objects which met the eye. The scene must have been the barrenness of desolation. Yet a good work was in progress. As the glacier slowly moved it ground into powder the rocks which impeded its progress, and formed that glacier mud which is now a rich soil for crops and fruit. The eater of the exquisite grapes, plums, and apples of Meran has to thank the glacier for them as well as the sun. The Polar climate and scenery of prehistoric times have given place to one of the healthiest and pleasantest climates within the temperate zone, and to a scenery of great variety and beauty.

Another revolution occurred in far later days, when history was written in another fashion than with ice upon the rocks. The valley was coveted and conquered by the Romans. The story is narrated in a condensed form by Professor Cölestin Stampfer in a small work published two years ago, and entitled "The Early History of Meran." Accepting the conclusions of Dr. Tappeiner in his study of the anthropology of Tyrol, Professor Stampfer questions whether the original inhabitants were either Celts or Etruscans, and he considers that they were a race apart, a race of a valiant and fierce character, which knew how to construct substantial stone fortresses without mortar, and to fight with intrepidity against the Romans. They were conquered, however, in the year 15 B.C. by Drusus. The young men were incorporated into the legions and sent to fight the battles of Rome in far distant lands. Roman settlers took the place of those who had been exiled or slain, and it is believed that they introduced the culture of the vine into this valley. The subjugation of this people, and the occupation of their land, was but a part of the plan of the Roman Emperor to form a highway from Italy to the Danube. A great trunk road, called the Via Claudia Augusta, was constructed, and a network of smaller roads was connected with it. Forts and places of refuge were erected at intervals along the roads, and the trader could pursue his vocation with ease and without fear. One of the largest of the fortresses was called Maja, and occupied the site upon which Obermais now stands. For two centuries after the Roman conquest the land enjoyed uninterrupted peace. The time came when the Romans were attacked and driven from the region which they had made to blossom like a garden. Germans took their places and profited by their labours. At the beginning of the present century the French essayed to repeat what the Romans had done before; their triumph was incomplete and evanescent; the fact of their presence in the land being chiefly kept alive by the memory of the deeds of the heroic Andreas Hofer, whom Bonaparte shot because he was a patriot. I said at the outset that Meran had attractions for persons of varied requirements and tastes; I have now written enough to indicate the directions in which careful study will reward those who sojourn here for their health's sake.

Meran has two suburbs—Untermais and Obermais—the former being lower down, the latter higher up, the valley. This gives a choice as to situation. The Curhaus is in Meran proper, and faces the principal promenade. It was built in 1871. A well-appointed bathing establishment forms a part of it. A compressed air bath, on the most approved principle, is largely used, under medical supervision, for the treatment of certain chest affections. A band of music plays twice daily, either in the open air or in the concert-room of the Curhaus. There is a theatre at Obermais. Those who enjoy lawn-tennis and skating can have plenty of both in winter. Of large hotels and fine villas there is no lack, and the shops are well supplied with goods. In addition to Roman Catholic churches a handsome German Protestant church was recently built. The services of the Church of England are held regularly during the season. Whether sufferers from advanced disease of the lungs should go to Meran is a matter for their medical advisers to decide. But invalids who have tried the Engadine would find as fine air, as much bright sunshine, and far more life and gaiety in Meran. Many sufferers from asthma find the relief there which other places have failed to yield. In short, those who are not very delicate, but who like to pass the winter in a pleasant and invigorating climate, might do worse than try Meran.

CHAPTER XI.

RONCEGNO.

Though many parts of Tyrol are as beaten ground as any part of Switzerland, yet there are not a few where the English-speaking tourist is rarely seen. The sightseers who overspread the Continent every year are familiar with the chief places on the railway which crosses the Brenner Pass, and forms an important line of communication between Germany, Austria, and Italy. It is probable that they have visited and admired Innsbruck, the capital of Tyrol. Botzen, the commercial capital, cannot be overlooked by them, as a stoppage must be made there on the way to and from Meran by rail. Large numbers visit Trent, the most important city in that region of Tyrol where the language of Italy is spoken by the inhabitants.

It would be a mistake for any tourist to pass Trent without stopping for a few days. As a fine specimen of a walled city it is noteworthy; the walls, which are in a good state of preservation, are of great antiquity, their builder being supposed to be Theodoric, King of the Ostrogoths. The Cathedral and many of the churches are striking examples of ecclesiastical architecture, whilst the Church of Santa Maria Maggiore was the one wherein the Council of Trent held its sittings between the years 1545 and 1563. It was hoped that this Council would promote the reformation of the Roman Catholic Church and the return of the Protestants into its fold. The portraits of those who took part in it, numbering upwards of 400, are preserved in a large painting, which has greater historic interest than artistic merit. A much more admirable monument is the historical work of Paolo Sarpi, whom Macaulay ranked at the head of Italian historians, who was one of Macaulay's favourites, and of whom he wrote in his diary that the "subject did not admit of vivid painting, but what Paolo Sarpi did he did better than anybody."

From Trent as a starting point, many places of great interest can be reached. One of these is Campiglio, where an "air-cure" can be had, and this place was much liked by the Empress Victoria when she was Crown Princess of Germany. She made a long sojourn at it with several of her children. Indeed, she and the good Emperor Frederick are amongst the few persons to whom the most picturesque parts of South Tyrol are familiar ground. The road to Roncegno, the place which I am about to describe, runs in the opposite direction. By following the road one arrives at Venice, and any one who does so is repaid by scenery far finer than that to be met with along the line of railway. After a drive of three hours after starting from Trent, one arrives at Roncegno.

When Professor Seegen and Dr. London told me at Carlsbad that the mineral water of Roncegno was one of the most remarkable with which they were acquainted, owing to the large quantity of arsenic contained in it, I made some inquiries about the place where this mineral water was produced. I found it no easy matter to obtain the desired information. I turned, but without success, to the last editions of "Murray," and "Baedeker," and the "Continental Bradshaw;" to Dr. Macpherson's "Baths and Wells of Europe," and Dr. Burney Yeo's "Climate and Health Resorts," without finding the particulars of which I was in quest. Roncegno is named in "Bradshaw's Dictionary of Mineral Waters and Health Resorts," and stated to be in Italy. In the map appended to that work, I found all the places mentioned in the text except Roncegno, and it was almost by accident that I learnt that it was about twenty miles from Trent, on the road to Venice, and that it was not in Italy, but in the Austrian Tyrol. Had the place been recently discovered and little frequented, I should not have felt surprise at the difficulty of procuring particulars about it. Yet it has been known as a watering-place for nearly thirty years, and upwards of 1000 invalids have visited and spent several weeks at it in one year. That in these circumstances it should not even be named in some guide-books to which many travellers on the Continent turn for information is certainly very strange. In giving a minute account of the place, I shall run no risk of repeating what is easily accessible and widely known.

Roncegno is situated in the valley of the Brenta, at the foot of Mount Tesobo, and at an elevation of 1700 feet above the level of the sea. High up on the mountain slope, at a time of which the exact date is unknown, mining was pursued, the mineral extracted from the ground being arsenical pyrites. In 1875 the mine was rediscovered, or rather was explored, and it was found to be of considerable extent. A central rail had been laid in the principal level, and a small wagon which ran upon it was found where the miners had left it. The visitors to Roncegno are in the habit of visiting this old mine, the sight being a curious one. The mine is a proof of the mountains in this region abounding in minerals being a fact well known to the inhabitants of the valleys and mountain slopes in bygone days, as far back, perhaps, as those when the Romans were lords of the country.

About thirty years ago the mineral water of Roncegno was discovered as the result of the observation of some peasants. They saw a golden-yellow liquid dripping from a fissure in the rock, and they observed that where it fell nothing would grow. What they saw became the subject of general talk, and Dr. Paoli, holding a post almost corresponding to that of an English parish doctor, was induced by what he heard to examine the strange liquid. He soon learnt that it was a strong mineral water, and that it was very rich in iron. He tried the effect of prescribing baths in it to patients who were suffering from debility and "pellagra," a malady which is common in these valleys and in all the southern regions where polenta is the principal food of the people. As the results were remarkable and satisfactory, Dr. Paoli communicated them to his colleagues. Arrangements were made with a view to the treatment being pursued in a more systematic way than in the house of each patient. A disused silk factory was converted into a bath-house, and the number of patients frequenting it soon became in excess of the accommodation. In 1860, a joint-stock company was formed, and a larger and better-arranged bath-house was constructed; but soon after it was found that the twenty baths in the new building were insufficient to meet the demand. Two other companies were formed successively to provide the capital required for building the present Curhaus, in which there are rooms for about 150 visitors, and baths for all those who are likely to need them. The grounds surrounding the Curhaus have been laid out and embellished, the roads have been improved, regular postal communication has been secured, while a telegraph office is open in the main building during the season. A few years ago the entire property passed into the hands of the Brothers Waiz, of Gradisca, who have spared no pains or expense to make it attractive. Indeed, I was surprised to find so large and well-arranged a building as the Curhaus at a place of which the guide-books in common use tell nothing, and of which the name is not to be found in some of the most recent maps. In addition to the accommodation supplied by the proprietors of the Curhaus, the visitor has the choice of rooms in five small hotels in the village of Roncegno.

Before proceeding to describe this place in greater detail, I may anticipate a question which will doubtless be on the lips of those who have read thus far—How comes it that a place of which so little appears to be known should be largely frequented by invalids, and be one well worth a visit by those who journey for change of scene? The simple answer is that many medical men of Austria and Northern Italy are well informed about Roncegno and its waters, and are in the habit of prescribing a course of the waters to their patients. Dr. Goldwurm, who has been the resident physician at the Curhaus in Roncegno for several years, has written a work on the subject which is included in the series of medical treatises on mineral baths and watering-places published by Herr Wilhelm Braumüller, of Vienna. In addition to this work, I have before me six treatises in Italian on the subject of Roncegno's baths and water, the first being dated 1873, and containing a chemical analysis of the mineral water, the last being dated 1884, and giving a description of the place itself and particulars of cures wrought there. Such is the explanation of what at first sight seemed a puzzle.

It is as well, perhaps, that the frequenters of Roncegno are sent there by their medical advisers, and are under medical supervision during their stay. The water is a potent medicine. At first it was used for bathing purposes only; now, however, the patient is ordered to drink as well as to bathe in it. As the dose is not more than two tablespoonfuls a day, diluted with plain water, it is clear that the water is considered more powerful than the mineral waters which are drunk in large quantities. Those who drink too much Roncegno water at one time, or continue taking it for too long a period, are soon made conscious of their error by suffering from oppression in the region of the stomach, loss of appetite, diarrhœa, smarting and twitching of the eyes.

Dr. Goldwurm complains that many patients leave the place after three weeks' sojourn, their belief being that they ought to have been cured if the water were really efficacious. It is very sensibly remarked by him that if an old and a young man suffer from the same malady, the course of treatment required in the case of the younger patient might be much shorter than in that of the elder. What Dr. Goldwurm protests against with emphasis, in common with his countrymen and colleagues who practise at an Austrian watering-place, is the impropriety of a patient who has been benefited by the treatment giving advice to others. At all Continental watering-places a strong desire prevails to dispense with the services of medical men, and the medical men naturally disapprove of each patient acting as his own doctor. Strict precautions are taken at Roncegno to prevent self-doctoring. Before a patient can begin a course of baths he or she is obliged to consult the resident physician. It is found easier, however, to enforce a medical consultation than to ensure that the advice given will be followed. This is exemplified in Dr.

Goldwurm's complaint that all patients think they may leave the place at the end of three weeks.

I can best exemplify the stringency with which visitors to the Curhaus are supervised, by translating and transcribing the Regulations, which are printed in Italian and German :

"1. Every stranger is requested to give his name and place of abode to the Director of the Bath-house, as well as those of his suite.

"2. The sum payable for inscribing any one's name is two florins.

"3. No stranger is allowed to begin a course of baths without having first consulted the physician attached to the establishment, whose first consultation is given free.

"4. A bath-room is at a bather's disposal for one hour only, and only for the hour fixed beforehand. Whoever fails to appear at the appointed time loses his turn, and he must either bathe at a later hour or do so in another room.

"5. Whoever wishes to bathe several times at the same hour daily is requested to provide himself with the requisite number of bathing tickets.

"6. The transfer of bathing tickets is permitted only after notification has been made at the office, and leave granted.

"7. The male and female bath-attendants are carefully-selected, and trusty, and trustworthy persons who are under the orders of a responsible manager; this is true also of the waiters and chambermaids, over whom a director or a matron is placed.

"8. The burning of a spirit-lamp for any purpose is forbidden in the private rooms.

"9. The honoured patients are requested not to make any noise, especially when people are in bed. Playing on the pianoforte is forbidden between eleven p.m. and nine a.m., and between noon and three p.m.

"10. All complaints are to be addressed to the Director."

The mineral water of Roncegno, as I have already said, is powerful in its action, hence the dose is small. Dr. Goldwurm is very particular as regards the way in which the dose is taken. If it should not exceed two tablespoonfuls it may be drunk off at a draught; but, if double that quantity be prescribed, then the patient is to sip the water. Those patients to whom the iron in the water will prove beneficial are ordered to drink it early on an empty stomach, and to walk for some time before eating; those, on the other hand, who take it on account of the arsenic are to do so immediately before breakfast, and then, after walking about for a time and taking a light repast, they are prepared for bathing in the water. Patients are warned against smoking, reading, and sleeping when in the bath, and they are recommended to keep moving and rubbing themselves while in the water.

It is noteworthy how careful the physicians at watering-places on the Continent are about their patients, and how minute they are in directing them what to do and what to avoid. A German and a French doctor resemble a German and a French policeman, in thinking that human beings are sure to go wrong unless they are kept in the right path by the heavy hand of authority. Great differences of opinion prevail as to whether a patient at Ronceguo should bathe twice in the same day. This appears to be a problem resembling that which divided the Big-endians from the Little-endians in the kingdom of Lilliput. In general, one bath daily is accounted enough, but in particular cases two may be beneficial. After arriving at this well-considered and common-sense conclusion, Dr. Goldwurm points out that Dr. Schivardi, an eminent Italian authority on balneology, is in the habit of prescribing two mineral water baths daily to the patients who visit Aqui, and, in addition, two mud baths. Though not disapproving of this heroic treatment, Dr. Goldwurm sagely concludes that the physician is alone competent to decide whether a patient should pass the greater part of the day in a bath, or whether he or she may bathe once and then trust that Nature will aid the mineral water in effecting a cure.

Besides drinking and bathing in the mineral water at Roncegno, the patients have another curative medium there in the form of a mud bath. But this bath differs in nearly all respects from the so-called mud baths at German and Austrian watering-places. The name is misleading, because the substance employed cannot accurately be termed "mud." At Carlsbad, Marienbad, and other places the substance which is loosely designated "mud" is really a mineralised peat or turf. At Roncegno the "mud" closely resembles yellow ochre. It is a deposit or sediment obtained from the tanks wherein the mineral water is stored. When steam is applied for a time it becomes semi-liquid, and in this form it is applied to the afflicted part of the human body. In peat or moor baths the patient is surrounded by the substance, just as in a bath of water; but the Roncegno mud bath is applied locally, much in the same way as a poultice. The mud poultice is said to be powerful in its effects, pimples soon covering the spot on which it has been placed. It is considered by Dr. Goldwurm to be very useful in cases of muscular rheumatism and chronic arthritis, in white swellings and sciatica. He states also that the eruption which appears when it is used does no injury, and quickly disappears. For other maladies several baths are provided, such as hot air, vapour, and douche baths. A room is set apart for inhaling the water in the form of spray, a mode of application which produces good results in diseases of the throat and air passages.

I am the more disposed to regard Roncegno water with favour, because it is not said to be a universal cure. Many mineral waters are lauded as highly as if they proceeded direct from the fabled fountain of perpetual youth, for which the early visitors to the New World sought with such eagerness, and sought in vain. Owing to being over-praised, these waters are classed by many persons in the category of quack medicines. None of the medical writers about Roncegno water profess that it will work miracles, but each of them maintains that its virtues are strikingly manifested when employed—first, in cases of anæmia, with its many and varied consequences; second, in many skin diseases; third, in malarial and intermittent fevers; fourth, in muscular rheumatism and inflammation of the joints; fifth, in chronic bronchial catarrh and incipient phthisis; and generally in all cases of exhaustion following a long illness. As this water is so little known, it may be useful to reproduce the analysis of its contents which was made by Professor Manetti, of the University of Pavia. For the convenience of readers who might not understand what was meant by kilogrammes of water, or how much a gramme represented, I shall state how many parts of the several mineral substances are contained in ten thousand parts of water:

Arsenic Acid	0·670
Ferric Oxide	20·400
Sulphuric Acid in combination	20·390
Sulphate of Ferrous Oxide	3·840
Sulphate of Cupric Oxide	0·270
Sulphate of Manganese	1·420
Sulphate of Ammonium	0·054
Sulphate of Aluminium	12·790
Sulphate of Magnesium	5·963
Sulphate of Calcium	8·300
Sulphate of Potassium	7·500
Chloride of Sodium	0·422
Carbonic Acid	0·049
Silica	2·910
Organic Matter	16·300
Total	101·278

The existence of a large proportion of arsenic is the distinguishing characteristic of Roncegno water, and its pre-eminence in this respect is apparent when the water is compared with well-known mineral waters in which arsenic is found. Of these, La Bourboule, in Auvergne, is the most noteworthy. While there are twenty-eight milligrammes of arseniate of soda in every litre of La Bourboule water, a corresponding quantity of Roncegno water contains sixty-seven, or nearly three times as much. Dr. Weiss, of the University of

Padua, who has written a pamphlet on the character and curative effect of the Roncegno water, maintains that many of the good results obtained from its use are due to the presence not only of arsenic, but also of manganese and iron in combination with it.

I have already said that the dose taken is not large, being from one or two tablespoonfuls daily; I may now add that the taste is not unpleasant when that quantity is diluted with water. For bathing purposes from one-fourth to one-third of mineral is added to the plain water. I took a bath, but did not find the sensation of a marked kind. I strictly observed the injunctions of the physician to the establishment, which are not to wear any kind of bathing dress, not to smoke, read, or sleep when in the bath, and always to keep the body in motion. I found it the easier to follow these injunctions, as I should never choose a mineral-water bath as a suitable place for smoking, reading, or sleeping.

Dr. Goldwurm, writing in 1884, gives an account of the growth in popularity of the baths and water at Roncegno, at which he had become the resident physician ten years before. When he first went there the number of bathers was 205; when he wrote it had increased to 922. He notes that among the visitors there were seven professors of medicine and twenty-eight practising physicians, of whom eight were undergoing treatment, the others being engaged in studying the water and the locality. It will be admitted, I think, that the mineral water which a medical man drinks must be regarded by him as an excellent medicine. A doctor's faith in the curative virtue of certain drugs or waters is generally strong enough to justify him in prescribing them, but it seldom suffices to make him take them himself. Whilst the number of patients at Roncegno has steadily increased, the demand for the water has risen also, 1,000 bottles being despatched in 1874 and 100,000 in 1884. Since Dr. Goldwurm thus wrote the increase has been continuous.

Patients who take up their abode in the Curhaus at Roncegno not only get medical advice, mineral water and baths under its roof, but they are also housed in comfort and fed abundantly. The proprietors hold out as an inducement to visitors that the food is well cooked and served without stint, "each dish being handed round more than once." I can confirm this statement, yet I must add that the fare is plain, and that the cooking is half Austrian and half Italian. A light and palatable red wine of the country is served at the table. It is doubtful, however, whether the supply of this wine will continue, as the vines have been attacked with a disease which threatens to render the vintage very poor. To all appearance the vines are healthy, and they are covered with grapes; but these grapes shrivel up towards the autumn instead of ripening. The failure of the vintage is a serious loss to the peasants, the cultivation of vines, mulberries, and maize being their principal occupation. Most of the peasants cultivate their own lands, and they are able to live comfortably. They speak Italian, or rather that dialect of it which is known as the Venetian.

Not far from Roncegno is the Tesino valley, which is filled with a curious population. The first settlers were immigrants from the Venetian provinces who tended flocks and herds. As their numbers increased they had to embrace other industries, with the result that they have come to be regarded as the chief manufacturers of the cheaper kinds of goods for which pedlars seek a market among the peasants and the poorer classes in all parts of the world. As soon as any native of the Tesino valley has acquired a small competency by trading in these articles, he returns home to spend his days in the place of his birth. The women generally remain behind to look after the sheep and cattle. As the men acquire a smattering of foreign languages during their wanderings, it happens that some inhabitant of the Tesino valley will be found who is acquainted with any European tongue.

About three miles from Roncegno lies the town of Borgo, on the bank of the Brenta. It is the principal one in the Sugana valley, and its population is between 4,000 and 5,000. In the old Roman days a military station was established there to guard the great road which ran between Tridentum and the Adriatic. At present the staple industry of Borgo is silk-weaving. The richer inhabitants have villas on the mountain slopes on either side of the wide and beautiful valley. High up in the mountains is Sella, a summer place of resort for those who wish to enjoy what is styled an "air-cure." The tourist who delights in ancient castles can have his taste gratified in the Sugana valley, there being as many as twenty, most of which are in ruins, but some are in good preservation and are inhabited, among them being Ivano, near Borgo.

For beauty of scenery and situation few spots outvie Roncegno, yet it is not to be recommended to those who merely wish to pass a pleasant holiday. The visitor who is not ailing is out of his element there. Those who enjoy it the most are those who may be said to mean business—in other words, they must visit it for what is styled "the cure." I cannot think that such persons will have any reason to complain of their accommodation and entertainment. They may find the life dull, the only relaxation being taking walks between baths and meals. On the other hand, their waking hours are fully occupied with the prescribed employment for regaining health. I might quote many cases, given in the works before me, of remarkable cures wrought at Roncegno; but I refrain from doing so, as the fact that one person has been benefited at a particular place furnishes no certain ground for concluding that another will be equally fortunate. The physicians of Germany and Austria study the characters of the several watering-places as much as they do the nature and operation of certain drugs, and thus they are enabled to order a patient to go to any one of these watering-places with as well-founded confidence as they write a prescription for an illness. Judging from the information which I have collected, I think that English physicians would do well to inform themselves about Roncegno and its arsenical-ferruginous water. Unless I err greatly, it seems clear that this water will act with remarkable benefit in all those maladies for which the mineral waters of Auvergne are in repute, and may even prove curative in many cases where the water of La Bourboule has failed to give relief.

The climate at Roncegno during the summer months is temperate and equable; indeed, the writers to whom I am indebted for many of the details which I have supplied, are unanimous in praising the climate as highly as the water. The season begins in May and closes at the middle of September. The director of the Curhaus, who resides there all the year round, says that in winter the weather is enjoyable; the sky being nearly always bright and the snowfall very trifling. Lofty mountains shelter Roncegno from the north. The Curhaus faces due south, and, as I have already written, the prospect is enchanting. The seeker after new places will not regret spending a short time in exploring the country around it. For the geologist the mountains abound in treasures. To any one who appreciates the beauties of Nature, the scenery is a perpetual treat; whilst, to the invalid for whose case the mineral water is suited, a sojourn at Roncegno ought to prove a pleasant and complete cure.

CHAPTER XII.

LEVICO.

At the entrance to the beautiful Sugana valley, on the high road from Trent to Bassano, and facing a picturesque lake, the small village of Levico is situated. The mineral water proceeding from Monte Fronte, at the base of which the village lies, has been in repute for two centuries, and Levico has long been frequented by invalids. Yet it is only of late years that it has attracted the sick and suffering from all quarters of the world. Even now Levico water is less known and valued in England and America than the mineral waters in many other parts of the Continent of Europe.

When describing Roncegno, I said that I had much trouble in ascertaining its situation, owing to the absence of information in the English guides to travellers abroad. I have found several references to Levico in books of travel; but I have failed to discover any adequate account of it in our language, the fullest particulars relating to it being contained in German and Italian works. I think that it deserves to be better known, though I fear that when it becomes more fashionable it will be less attractive. A health resort which the ordinary tourist never visits has generally a charm of its own. A crowded and very fashionable watering-place is one to be avoided by those who wish to enjoy themselves. There is no fear of Levico being overrun with tourists so long as it remains inaccessible by railway. At present the visitor has to leave the railway at Bassano or Trent in order to reach it. There is a project, indeed, of making a railway through the Sugana Valley; but for years to come, it will probably be necessary to spend several hours in a diligence or carriage in order to reach Levico. The ordinary tourist and sightseer prefers places on the railway to those on the high road.

Travellers on the Continent who are tired of the regular round and beaten path will find much that is fresh and interesting in the less explored valleys of the Austrian Tyrol, and they will experience a new and pleasant sensation in walking, riding, or driving along the romantic road which runs between Trent and Bassano. The view is beautiful throughout. Not long after leaving Trent the gorge of the Fersina is reached, and a more impressive spectacle than the cascade which dashes down from the highest point cannot be seen elsewhere. The road itself recalls the Corniche between Nice and Mentone, and some parts of the new road by the sea between Nice and Monaco. At certain places, the rock out of which the road is hewn overhangs it and has a menacing aspect of insecurity. At the highest point, and adjoining the cascade, there is a fortification from which cannon are pointed so as to command the road in each direction, and it seems clear that any body of men coming along the confined passage would be swept away by a well-directed fire. On the other hand, it is improbable that any commander of troops would take them along a road where they would certainly be shot down before they could attack the fortifications.

About half-way between Trent and Levico is the small town of Pergine, on the left bank of the river Fersina. Silk-weaving is the chief industry of the inhabitants. In situation and appearance Pergine reminded me of Stirling, the principal town at the entrance to the Scottish Highlands, the castle which dominates Pergine having a great external resemblance to that of Stirling. This one belongs to the Bishop of Trent, who seems to give no heed to its maintenance, as it is rapidly falling into decay, the walls sheltering a few poor peasants. From a distance it seems in perfect preservation, and if the reality be less pleasing on near approach, the state of neglect in the interior does not mar the view from the walls. Conspicuous in the landscape are the strange mountain summits of the dolomite formation, some being entirely denuded of vegetation, others being covered with wood. Whilst the river Fersina courses down one valley, the lakes Caldanazzo and Levico fill and adorn another. They are divided by an elevation called Monte Brenta, and the river Brenta, which has its source in them, flows along the valley for twenty-one miles till it falls into the Adriatic at Brondolo. Though Pergine is more pleasantly situated than Levico, yet the latter has the special advantage of being sheltered from cold winds, and of possessing an equable climate; hence it is the better fitted as a place of sojourn for invalids.

Levico is probably as little known as Roncegno to the English and American frequenters of Continental health resorts. I think that it deserves more attention than it has received, judging from the particulars which I collected on the spot. I have already said that its mineral water was famous two centuries ago. Two springs were then turned to account; the stronger one was employed for the production of sulphate of iron, the weaker one for drinking purposes, both being now used for alleviating or curing many maladies. It was not till the end of the last century that the medicinal virtue of the water received adequate recognition. The first bath-house was erected in 1814. In 1816 the use of the stronger of the two springs was forbidden by the Government authorities, after Dr. Pinali, of Trent, had discovered and reported that the water contained arsenic. However, permission to use the water as a medicine was granted when it was found that some persons who drank it in moderation were not poisoned, but, on the contrary, were cured of their ailments. Since then the arsenic has made it prized and famous. The proprietors of the Levico mineral water boast that no other one is so rich in this popular poison; the proprietors of the Roncegno water make the same boast. I have tried to ascertain which is in the right, with the result of finding it impossible to reconcile the conflicting evidence. As the chief importance of both mineral waters consists in their arsenical-ferruginous character, it may save other inquirers some trouble if I give the conclusions at which, after a careful inquiry and consideration of all the facts, I have arrived regarding them.

It is scarcely necessary to say that a keen rivalry exists between Levico and Roncegno; they are close together, and the inhabitants of the one seem to think it wrong to admit that any good mineral water can proceed from the other. A like jealousy exists between Carlsbad and Marienbad. The water of some springs in each is almost identical, the only difference being that in the one it is warm, and in the other cold; but the stranger who asks a native of Carlsbad what he thinks of the mineral water at Marienbad, or a native of Marienbad what he thinks of that at Carlsbad, will be assured that the water about which he asks is the one to be avoided. Rival watering-places resemble rival beauties in their inability to do justice to each other's merits; it may be added with perfect truth that they are both eager and accustomed to speak evil one of another. In Dr. Weiss's small work upon Roncegno, it is said that, while the Roncegno water contains sixty-seven milligrammes of arsenic to the litre, that of La Bourboule contains fourteen, and Levico little more than one only. He makes the mistake of saying that Levico is in Italy, whereas, like Roncegno, its near neighbour, it is in the Austrian Tyrol. Perhaps he underestimates the quantity of arsenic in La Bourboule water, though the figures which he gives correspond with those published in Dr. Macpherson's "Baths and Wells of Europe." On the other hand, Dr. Burney Yeo, in his "Climate and Health Resorts," represents La Bourboule water as containing twenty-eight milligrammes of arsenic to the litre. The proprietors of the Levico water have published an analysis of it made by Professor L. Barth and Dr. H. Weidel, of Vienna, according to which it appears that the proportion of arsenic in it is not one milligramme to the litre, as stated by Dr. Weiss, but is ninety milligrammes. The Viennese chemists style Levico water unique of its kind. The figures which they cite justify them in so doing, yet they might have been more comprehensive in their comparisons. They show how much richer in arsenic Levico water is as compared with the waters of Wiesbaden and Rippoldsau, which are known to contain but little, and they omit to notice the stronger and more noteworthy arsenical water of La Bourboule. I have said enough to show how difficult it is to obtain precise details on this head.

The seeker after knowledge will have another stumbling-block to surmount should he obtain and read the work on Levico by Dr. Joseph Pacher. He was physician there for upwards of ten years. His small work, which was published at Vienna in 1873, has long been the authentic guide to Levico. At the end of it he gives an analysis of the water made by Professor Manessi, which shows the quantity of arsenic to be not much more than a trace. It is possible, of course, that the later analysis of Professor Barth is the more correct of the two, or it may be that the water tested in each case varied in strength. Either explanation is plausible; but the fact remains that no reader of all the printed documents about Levico or Roncegno can be quite certain what to believe.

Having impartially set forth the case as I find it, I may assume that no mineral water now known is stronger in arsenic than that of Levico, and I may add that if the figures I have quoted, which give La Bourboule as containing twenty-eight, Roncegno sixty-five, and Levico ninety milligrammes to the litre, are thoroughly trustworthy, then there can be no question as to the fact. Certainly, I have learnt enough about the Levico water to admit that it is a remarkable one, and well deserving the notice of our chemists and physicians. In Austria no doubt is entertained by those who are competent to form an opinion that this mineral water is noteworthy. The Minister of the Interior sent Dr. Preiss to investigate it in 1857, and his report was to the effect that few mineral springs were more curious than that of Levico, and that the Levico water had great therapeutic power.

The mineral springs in Levico belong to the commune or parish, from which a company has leased them. The weaker spring has always been communal property; the stronger one was acquired from the Dorna family early in the century for a sum equal to £40 sterling; it would not be sold now for £40,000.. Neither spring is in Levico itself, each springing from the mountain side at Vitriolo, at an elevation of 4500 feet. At this height a bathing establishment is open for a short time in the year, some patients preferring to drink the water and bathe in it at the source, and at the same time to enjoy the advantage of breathing mountain air. Dr. Elia Sartori, the present physician to the bathing establishment at Levico, who has written an account, in Italian, of the springs and the place, states in the course of it that Vitriolo is growing in popularity, and that it is destined to become notable amongst Alpine health resorts. Vitriolo is reached from Levico on donkey-back in about three hours. The view from it is extensive and enchanting, yet it is questionable whether any one but a person in search of health would care to spend three weeks at this sequestered and very quiet spot. A medical man resides in the bath-house at Vitriolo during the season. Those who wish for further professional advice must summon a doctor from Levico. For making a special visit the doctor is entitled to a fee of six florins, which seems a very small remuneration considering that at least six hours are spent in ascending and descending the mountain. At Levico, however, this charge is thought high, as the payment for an ordinary visit there is one florin only. Though such a fee seems a miserable pittance from an English and American point of view, yet it is large compared with that which, according to Smollett, was the authorised charge at

Nice when he was there in 1764. He records that the Nice physicians then received a sum equivalent to sixpence for each visit, and that even this small sum was given with a grudge.

The village of Levico does not differ in appearance from the majority of Tyrolese towns of a corresponding size. It is difficult to say how many inhabitants it has. I have read that they number between 3000 and 4000, and I have also read in the work of Dr. F. G. de Massarellos that they are as many as 7000. In that work it is also said that two small silk factories there give employment to a considerable number of persons; that two advocates and one notary represent the legal profession; that two physicians and two apothecaries help to keep the people in good health and to smooth their latter end; and that there are nine common schools, attended by 850 children. The most striking edifice is the church, which is a new building in the Lombardo-Byzantine style, and it is far more pleasing to the eye than the churches in this valley, which resemble Roman temples more closely than Christian churches. In addition to the Curhaus, where about 100 visitors can be accommodated, there are eight hotels and three villas for their reception. When I add that between 2,000 and 3000 persons were under treatment last season—in other words, spent not less than three weeks in

BATHING UNDER DIFFICULTIES. 251

Levico—it will be admitted that a place so largely frequented should not be overlooked, as has hitherto been the case, by English writers on Continental health resorts.

Patients under treatment at Levico are ordered to take baths regularly as well as to drink the water. The bather in the mineral water is said to be invigorated. He certainly experiences a new sensation. Though not under treatment, I was permitted to pay the usual charge and to take a bath. This exceptional privilege was granted after I had stated that I was actuated by curiosity and did not mind the risk of bathing in Levico mineral water. The rule is that those who are allowed to bathe at all must bathe a certain number of times, and do so in compliance with the orders of the physician attached to the establishment. The mineral water descends about 4000 feet from its mountain source, and during its progress a marked change takes place in its appearance. When it issues from the ground at Vitriolo it is limpid and colourless; when it enters a bath at Levico it resembles port wine. The mere colour of the water is unimportant; but its astringent properties are not only marked, but they are sometimes painful unless precautions have been adopted. Dr. Sartori advises the patients whose skins are tender and sensitive, either to apply vaseline before entering the water or else to bathe in plain water after leaving the bath. If this advice be disregarded, then the patients will pay the penalty in the shape of great cutaneous irritation. Thus they will learn by painful experience that Levico water is too strong to be trifled with.

Those who drink the water are recommended to exercise moderation. A wineglassful daily of the stronger water is a full dose; a larger quantity of the weaker water may be mixed with wine and imbibed at meals. Dr. Massarellos, who practises at Munich, writes that he is in the habit of prescribing Levico water to his patients, and that they take it along with their beer at dinner and supper. He adds that the beer does not taste any the worse for the addition, and that the action of the water is quite as marked when it is taken in this way as when drunk alone.

The late Dr. Pacher and Dr. Sartori, who has succeeded him as resident physician, generally agree as to the way in which the treatment at Levico is to be pursued. Both hold that no one is to begin the "cure" who is not advised to do so by a medical man; in fact, the patient who wishes to be his own doctor finds that he cannot succeed, as the use of the baths is forbidden to patients who are unprovided with a medical certificate. At the outset the bath is composed of two-thirds plain and one-third mineral water; towards the end of the course these proportions are reversed, as by that time the body is supposed to be fitted for immersion in mineral water very slightly diluted. The temperature of the water, according to Dr. Pacher, should range from 82° to 86° Fahrenheit; Dr. Sartori prefers that the temperature should range from 91° to 95°, and both hold that no bather should remain longer than half an hour in the water. With that minute and exasperating attention to detail which is characteristic of some Austrian medical men, Dr. Pacher is careful to point out that the patient should ascertain whether the water is at the proper temperature, and that he should do this either by testing it with a thermometer or else by putting his foot in the water and judging by his feelings. He is also copious and wearisome in enforcing the propriety of carefully drying the whole body after leaving the bath—this being a matter which no one, I should think, is likely to neglect. It is possible, however, that unless warned to the contrary, some of Dr. Pacher's patients omitted drying their bodies after stepping out of a bath and before putting on their clothes. Dr. Sartori is equally careful in enjoining upon bathers the necessity of drying themselves, while he further advises, as I have said already, that they should anoint themselves with vaseline before entering the water.

The medical men who have written about Levico water praise it on account of its containing the requisite proportions of iron, copper, and arsenic. As Dr. Massarellos puts it—the arsenic stimulates the secretions, the copper soothes the nerves, the iron strengthens the blood. At Roncegno, where the water has a close general resemblance to that of Levico, the cures wrought are ascribed to its containing, in due proportions, arsenic, iron, and manganese. Very little is thought of the copper at Roncegno and as little at Levico of the manganese. At both places the patients are well fed as well as well dosed. Dr. Sartori sagely remarks that the most suitable diet is that which agrees the best with a patient. Writing, not as a patient but as a critic, I should pronounce the food provided at the Curhaus, where I had the pleasure of making Dr. Sartori's acquaintance, to be too rich for those who have not very good digestions. Perhaps there is nothing more difficult to settle than the appropriate diet for patients at a Continental watering-place. So long as they all come from the same country the matter is easy enough; but when people of various nationalities congregate in order to be cured, then the problem becomes serious. At some watering-places, such as Marienbad and Carlsbad, where the regimen is half the cure, it has been found necessary to revise the rules laid down many years ago. In the early days of these health resorts their frequenters came from Austria, Germany, and Russia. Of late years they have been frequented by English, Americans, French, and Italians also. Now the food eaten at home by these persons differs as much as the languages spoken by each. The medical man at a watering-place should not only be able to speak many tongues, but he should be versed in the domestic habits and the personal constitutions of many peoples. At Levico the necessity for an acquaintance with international medicine has not yet arisen. The majority of the visitors come from Italy, and they are as ready to enjoy the dishes of their native land as they are to speak its language. Few persons in Levico speak or understand German. The visitor who is unversed in Italian will find a difficulty in having his wishes gratified. As yet the polyglot hotel porter, who speaks many tongues fluently and imperfectly, is an unknown personage in Levico, the visitors being expected to act as their own interpreters.

Dr. Pacher says that the treatment at Levico forms a good "after-cure" for those who have been at a watering-place in other parts of Austria. The maladies for which the water is said to be best adapted are those of which anœmia is the basis or cause, and it is specially suited for the treatment of a large class of female ailments. The proportion of women to men undergoing the cure at Levico is as three to one. At Vitriolo men are in the majority. Delicate children of both sexes derive great benefit from the Levico baths and waters. Dr. Sartori states that the invalids to whom these baths and waters will afford no relief are those suffering from acute fever, from serious heart disease, or who are in an advanced stage of pulmonary consumption. He is most comprehensive, however, in designating the class of persons who should visit Levico for treatment. He advises all who are ailing but not really ill to try Levico in order that they may not grow worse, while he is convinced that those who have been ill but are not quite recovered, and that those who are afflicted with some disease of which they wish to get rid, should follow their example.

The amusements provided for patients are few and simple, consisting chiefly in taking walks, fishing in the lake, and listening to the band which plays twice weekly on the terrace in front of the Curhaus. Dr. Massarellos is emphatic in recommending all patients who visit Levico to leave their cares at home. The advice is good and old. It was given to the ancient

Romans, as is shown by the following inscription over a famous Roman bath: "Leave care behind if you would depart in health; care hinders cure." The mineral springs at this place may contain the exact proportion and quantity of iron, arsenic, and copper necessary for relieving many forms of illness, yet the sick and afflicted who have a right to count upon deriving the greatest benefit from a sojourn at Levico must be in a frame of mind suitable for profiting by the medicinal virtues of the mineral waters.

CHAPTER XIII.

ARCO.

THE health resorts in the vast Austro-Hungarian Empire number about 350. As not less than a week or ten days spent on the spot is sufficient time during which to learn the peculiarities and attractions of each, many years would be required to make an adequate examination of them all, and several volumes could be filled with the results of such an investigation. Those of which an account is given in the present work have been selected because they are either popular and well known by name, or else because they are not known in England and America, yet deserve to be visited.

I may assume, I think, that Arco is as unfamiliar to English and American sojourners on the Continent of Europe as Roncegno and Levico. It is a noteworthy place, occupying in Austrian estimation the position which is held in Italy by San Remo and in France by Mentone. Every place wherein invalids or delicate persons can pass the winter in comparative comfort is a subject of curiosity to a large class on both sides of the Atlantic. It is enough to cause Arco to excite general interest to say that it is one of these places, and that its advocates are enthusiastic about its future.

Before visiting Arco I could learn little about it in any other book than the small one from the pen of Dr. Gustav von Kottowitz, which was published in Vienna five years ago. In Arco itself I obtained two other treatises concerning it, the one being entitled *Der Klimatische Curort Arco*, by Dr. Eduard Leisching, the other *Arco und die Riviera als Winterstationen für Lungenkranke*, by Dr. H. A. Ramdohr, late staff-surgeon in the Saxon army. Both of those named are dated 1886. Besides these and other less important works, I have before me a copy of a pamphlet issued by the authorities there, and entitled " Arco : Autumn and Winter Climatic Resort." What I read before visiting Arco made me desirous of seeing it. I am pleased to have made the visit, as I have found much that was attractive in the place, though I did not find it quite so perfect as it is depicted. Indeed, most places are either more or less charming in reality than upon paper; the beauties of Nature may defy description, but the pleasures due to a fine climate depend upon accident. A single wet or gloomy day upsets preconceived notions about a given place being a new

Lotus land. If a second Garden of Eden were described in the exaggerated style used by the eulogists of certain health resorts, it might disappoint expectation when actually visited.

Arco is less than four miles distant from Riva, at the head of Lake Garda, and about ten miles from Mori, on the line of railway between Botzen and Verona. It may be reached by coach from Trent, as well as from Riva and Mori. It is situated on the right bank of the River Sarca, which falls into Lake Garda at Torbole. The valley in which it lies is shut in on all sides but the south with mountains rising from four to seven thousand feet, and the northern opening, through which the river runs, is blocked by a mass of rock 370 feet high, upon which stands the ruined castle of the Counts of Arco. This mass breaks the current of wind from the north. Another elevation, called Monte Brione, lessens the force of the wind blowing from the opposite direction. Thus Arco is sheltered from strong blasts, its almost windless character being one of its chief boasts and attractions. It is noted also as a place where little rain falls. Yet, though the air be still and dry, there is no sensation of closeness, as is the drawback in many mountain valleys. The Sarca valley is spacious enough both for air and locomotion, its length being about four miles and the breadth about three. All the ground is under cultivation. Not a morsel of it is left untilled between Arco and Riva, the crops being grapes, maize, and mulberries, and as the maize and mulberries are cultivated between the rows of vines, the aspect is that of a most fruitful and prolific land. On the slopes behind the houses there are hundreds of olive trees, and the olive oil expressed from the fruit is said to be of excellent quality. It is rather hastily inferred that the presence of olive trees is a sign that the climate is very mild. Now, olive trees flourish near Avignon, in Provence, yet the winters at Avignon are not balmy. It is probable that a low temperature is less felt at Arco than in less sheltered spots, and thus it may be a pleasant place in the winter time even when the temperature is not high.

Dr. Ramdohr's account of Arco in winter has an exceptional value. He was there from the middle of January till the middle of February, and he was an invalid suffering from chronic disease of the throat and chest. He was a medical critic as well as a patient, and his criticisms have a value unattainable by those of a sufferer who is not also a physician. Any patient is ready enough to find fault, but no patient who is devoid of professional training can speak or write with authority. Other writers about Arco record that snow seldom falls there, and that when snow does fall it melts almost immediately. Dr.

Ramdohr was in Arco when snow fell in abundance. According to him the snow melted but slowly, although the sun shone brightly the day following the heavy fall, the reason being that there was frost every night. The snow remained on the ground for a fortnight in places which the sunshine did not reach. In Dr. Ramdohr's opinion, this was a proof that the climate of Arco was unlike such a southern one as could be found and enjoyed on the Riviera. Though he is quite right so far, his conclusion ought not to be accepted without qualification. Snow falls in Meran during the winter, yet many invalids are benefited by residing there. Snow falls in the Engadine, and skating is common there, yet many invalids whose chests are delicate pass the winter in the Engadine not only in comparative comfort, but with great advantage. I was greatly impressed by the statement of an informant who had passed several winters at San Remo and Mentone before spending one in Arco. His verdict was that, though the climate on the Riviera was warmer, it was less pleasant than that of Arco on the whole, chiefly because the latter place enjoyed an almost complete immunity from wind storms. There is no doubt that the violent winds which rage along the Riviera in winter are trying as well as disagreeable to invalids, and, if the air be so still at Arco during the winter months as every one says it is, then it has a great natural pre-eminence over many winter resorts farther south. Dr. Ramdohr complains that the air was too still to please him. In March and April, when most of the invalids take their departure, there is the maximum of wind.

Dr. von Kottowitz, who, as a practising physician at Arco during the winter, naturally notes everything in its favour, is glad to point out how much more agreeable the temperature is there than at Meran. For four occasions on which the thermometer marked a degree or more below freezing point in January at Arco, it marked several degrees below freezing point on twenty at Meran. He also notes with satisfaction that skating, which is a winter's amusement at Meran, cannot be practised at Arco. Writers about Meran are careful to note that invalids can skate there in their shirt-sleeves, delighting in frost and sunshine at the same time. Doctors at a health resort have an irresistible tendency to conclude that their patients ought to appreciate physic in whatever form it is presented to them. Both in Meran and Arco provision is made against the cold; the bedrooms, even those facing the south, have double windows, while not only are the halls and passages of the best hotels warmed by hot air, but there is a porcelain stove in every room. It is chiefly in the evening and the early morning that the need for artificial warmth is felt, and there is enough sunshine during the day to permit of a delicate person sitting out of doors. On the Riviera the houses are imperfectly provided with heating appliances, the result being that when the sun is obscured for days together, which sometimes happens, or when water freezes, which is no rarity, the invalids wintering there suffer terribly from the cold.

Statistics drawn from observations extending over ten years show that the invalid at Arco can count upon spending several hours a day in the open air. During these hours it is assumed that the sun shines and that the conditions are suitable for walking or sitting out of doors, the early morning and the hours after sunset being excluded from the calculation. It appears, then, that the invalid's day, as it is called, is nine hours long in October, seven in November, six in December, five in January, six in February, eight in March, and the whole time between sunrise and sunset in April.

Dr. Ramdohr, who visited both Arco and the Riviera for his health's sake, is of opinion that invalids are commonly and improperly treated as hot-house plants. In the cases of patients whose lives can be prolonged for a short time only, and that by the exercise of the greatest care, it is right, he thinks, to take every possible precaution; but he holds that in the cases of others, whose condition is such that a complete cure may be effected, there ought to be less restriction as to walking out at all times and in all weathers. He says that he tried the experiment of being constantly in the open air and found that it answered perfectly; he contrasts his experience with that of those who, when the weather is threatening or unpleasant, spend the whole day within doors in close, ill-ventilated, and unhealthy rooms. He admits that he formerly believed in the importance of invalids not venturing out except when the weather was considered favourable; but now he urges, as the result of personal experience, the advisability of regular exercise in the open air every day, unless on the very rare occasions when it would be injurious for a person in good health to venture out. One drawback of the Riviera is the prevalence of strong winds; another is the superabundance of dust. Dr. Ramdohr enlarges on the dust plague, and he condemns several places on account of its prevalence. At Arco, however, it is almost unknown. No traffic is allowed in the street where the principal hotels and villas are situated; the wind is seldom strong in winter, and the clouds of dust which sweep along the streets of Mentone, Nice, and Cannes are unknown at Arco.

At Arco, as at Meran, the invalids who elect

to pass the winter have other curative arrangements at their disposal than clear air and bright sunshine. German and Austrian physicians have a great belief in baths as methods of cure, and where nature has not provided mineral water at a health resort, artificial means are taken to supplement the deficiency. There is an establishment at Arco wherein baths of all kinds are provided, exclusive of those which are required for the application of what is styled the hydropathic system. A consumptive patient is seldom benefited, and is often sent with greater rapidity to his grave, by being subjected to the cold water cure. For those who wish to try the experiment without fear of the inevitable result, the provision of hydropathic appliances is as complete as can be wished. Patients suffering from forms of throat disease, which the most enthusiastic advocate of cold water applications does not profess to treat, have other forms of cure at their service. These embrace and include various kinds of medicated inhalations. Compressed air baths, from which asthmatic patients sometimes obtain great relief, are also obtainable, while those who require to be treated through the medium of electricity can have their wish gratified. This bath-house is admirably arranged, and it must prove serviceable to many invalids by placing within the power of their medical advisers methods of treatment or cure which are superior to drugs, and form a supplement to fine air and bright sunshine. It is noteworthy that while at any Austrian health resorts to which invalids are sent to pass the winter months, a large bath-house is regarded as an indispensable adjunct, no corresponding arrangement prevails at the winter homes on the Riviera. If the same attention were paid to this important form of hygiene by the authorities at the notable places on the Riviera from San Remo to Hyères, the physicians who practise in these health resorts for invalids might be able to boast of effecting more cures. It is possible, however, that too much trust is placed in baths at Austrian health resorts, and that too much confidence is shown throughout Southern Italy and France in the curative influences of sunshine and soft air. A judicious combination of the two is obviously the golden mean.

In the English translation of a German pamphlet about Arco issued by a committee chosen to make its advantages known, and render it attractive to invalids, it is said that "Arco is well suited as a residence for persons suffering from affections of the chest and throat, from want of blood, want of appetite, rheumatism, gout, paralysis, nervousness, chronic catarrh of the stomach, intermittent fever;

also for those recovering from illness or disposed to consumption, for weakly, scrofulous, rickety children." From this it will be seen that many persons are included among the number of those who will benefit by a sojourn at Arco. Nine medical men practise there during the winter, and two apothecaries dispense medicines all the year round. One of the forms of treatment regularly carried out there is scarcely known in England; it has been devised by Professor Oertel and it is called the *Terrain Cur*. I fancy that some persons would translate this "earth cure," and they might be excused for doing so, and also for supposing that it referred to a method of partial burial in the ground like that which has been practised at different times and places. But the clumsy and obscure phrase has quite another meaning, and it implies a mode of treatment by taking walks. Walking about for the sake of one's health is nothing very new; but, then, German physicians are skilled in turning an old thing to a new account and proclaiming that they have made a discovery. Patients, it must be admitted, take kindly to old things under fresh aspects. Tell an invalid to walk for an hour daily, and he will not greatly value the advice; but tell him to try the *Terrain Cur*, and he will gladly make the experiment, though all he does is to walk for a stated time. In order that this form of treatment may be conducted with a due regard for appearances, the principal walks around Arco, as at other places where the *Terrain Cur* is in vogue, are carefully numbered. Coloured signboards at every turning serve to indicate each particular walk. It is said that by this classification and regulation of the walks, the suitable amount of exercise can be prescribed to and taken by a patient, that the weak are not likely to over-exert themselves, and the strong are as little likely to suffer from insufficient muscular exertion. It is said, moreover, that many forms of illness can be successfully treated in this fashion. What is beyond doubt is that the *Terrain Cur* gives a medical man an additional hold upon his patient. Besides enjoining upon a patient what he is to drink, eat, and avoid, what medicine he is to swallow, and what hours he is to keep, where and how he is to live, the physician who prescribes the *Terrain Cur* can also exercise a strict control over his walks abroad.

The committee which acts at Arco in the interests of the visitors is a body almost unknown at some health resorts elsewhere, and is never heard of at such places in England or America. Its functions and its constitution deserve to be better known, and, as I have before me a copy of the statutes governing that of Arco, I may extract from it the salient and more interesting points. It is necessary for a place to be authoritatively recognized as a health resort before such a committee can be formed, and after a place ceases to be so recognized then the committee ceases to exist. At Arco the committee consists of eight persons, who serve for three years, the *podesta*, or mayor, being one and acting as chairman. The duties of the committee are defined as consisting in—firstly, doing everything that is required for attracting visitors to Arco; secondly, improving the place generally and rendering it more agreeable to the public, supporting and encouraging musical performances and other kinds of amusement; thirdly, publishing advertisements and causing articles to be inserted in newspapers; fourthly, providing for the supply of German physicians; fifthly, arranging for the collection and employment of the tax upon visitors and others who are liable to pay it; sixthly, encouraging the grape, milk, and whey cure; seventhly, settling disputes between visitors and the inhabitants; eighthly, doing whatever may be required to render the place more popular as a health resort. I need not reproduce the minute directions which are laid down for carrying out these objects. It is sufficient to add that each visitor who stays longer than four days is bound to contribute two florins a month to the fund at the disposal of this committee, that children under twelve pay half that sum, and the servants of visitors one-fourth. The poor who can show that their means will not permit of any payment are exempted from taxation. As the result of this arrangement, such a place as Arco is rendered much more attractive than it would otherwise be; a good band of music plays daily for the delectation of those who have nothing better to do than to listen; whilst the grounds and public gardens are kept in excellent order. If no such committee existed the visitors would have frequent occasion to complain; owing to the action of such a committee many persons are attracted to Arco. Had it not been for the documents issued by the committee, one of which fell into my hands, I might not have visited it.

I think that the account which I have given of the existence and action of such a committee may be fitly supplemented with a useful moral. In England there are several places which have as genial a climate in winter as Arco, Meran, and many of the small towns on the Riviera. Yet they are little known, and as places of residence they lack the attractions which gratify invalids. A small sum of money expended in making them better known and better worth visiting would be speedily and amply repaid by an influx of visitors. I refrain from mentioning names; but I assert with confidence that from the Isle of Wight to Penzance there are eight health resorts which only require a little judicious supervision and notice to become quite as popular among those who wish to forget the winter months amid bright sunshine and blooming flowers without leaving their native land. A little organisation on the Austrian model would make many English health resorts as much appreciated as they deserve to be.

Though Arco has been officially recognised as a health resort for fifteen years only, it is better known in Germany, Austria, and Russia, and is more frequented by persons from those countries, than many places of much older date. This is chiefly due, perhaps, to the fact of persons of high position by birth having been among its earliest frequenters. When writing about Meran, I stated how much more popular it became after the Empress of Austria had passed a winter there. Nice owes much of its popularity to the fact of crowned heads or heirs to crowns being in the habit of visiting it. Now, Arco had the good fortune to attract the notice of his Imperial Highness the Archduke Albert, commander-in-chief of the Austrian army, who built a commodious house, laid out the surrounding grounds in a beautiful style, and who has spent the winter months there for some time back. The Crown Prince of Austria has visited it, as have the Queen of Bavaria, the King and Queen of Saxony, and many Imperial and Royal

Highnesses. Where they go others gladly follow; hence Arco's rapid rise and extending fame.

I am glad to have seen Arco before it was transformed, if not injured, by prosperity. Very few health resorts are improved by becoming fashionable. Torquay, one of the best in England, was far more attractive, thirty years ago, when it was still a small town of villas, and was not, as it now is, overgrown and overbuilt. When the first winter visitors went to Mentone in 1855 they may have found the place less attractive in some respects than at present, but there is little doubt that it was far healthier, as the sewage problem did not then vex the minds of the inhabitants. When Smollett visited Nice, upwards of a century ago, that Italian city was a very different one from the existing French one; but it is doubtful whether it was not a pleasanter place of sojourn. Since Lord Brougham caused Cannes to be changed from a small and neglected fishing village into a large aggregation of sumptuous hotels and villas, there has been no perceptible increase in the charms which made him select it as a place of abode. Monte Carlo, which is now styled "the beauty-spot of the Riviera," better deserved the title when it was half its present size, and when olive, orange, and lemon trees covered the spaces which are now crowded with houses.

Building is going on rapidly at Arco; the prettiest open spaces and best situations are in process of being covered with villas. Should the present rate of increase in the houses continue, the place will soon be entirely ruined. There, as at other places of the kind, every new house causes a twofold injury. In the first place, the rude sanitary arrangements at present prevailing are rendered still more imperfect and dangerous as house is added to house; in the second, the area which is covered with houses is so much ground abstracted from the space where the air is kept sweet and wholesome. As land is not costly, and as villas can be erected very cheaply at Arco, there is but small chance of the plague of over-building being stayed.

Judging from my own observation, and from the testimony which I have collected, I should pronounce Arco a pleasant place wherein to spend the winter months. It is improbable that those who are in an advanced stage of consumption can derive that benefit there which is unprocurable elsewhere. For those who are very sensitive to cold it may be less suitable than some parts of the Riviera, or than Egypt, Algeria, and Madeira. Yet, to the large class who spend a part of the winter in the South of Europe because they wish to enjoy a more genial climate than that of London, and who are delicate but not seriously ill, a sojourn at Arco can be confidently recommended. For such visitors it would have the charm of novelty as well as other attractions. The season begins on the 1st of September and ends on the 1st of May. Enthusiastic writers may exaggerate and mislead readers in depicting Arco as an earthly paradise. Still, if but a part of what they say in its praise be well-founded, it resembles paradise during the winter months quite as closely as any reasonable person should expect to find in that part of the habitable globe which is included within the vast Empire of Austria.

CHAPTER XIV.

ABBAZIA.

The Austrian Riviera extends between Lovrana and Volosca, at the head of the Gulf of Fiume, and Abbazia is a spot near Volosca which is largely frequented for its sea bathing in the summer and autumn months and for its mild climate in the winter. About ten years ago, when I was at Fiume in the dead of winter, and heard much said in praise of Abbazia, I visited it. What I then saw entirely confirmed all that I had been told.

Upwards of a century ago, Balthasar Hacquet, a medical man who travelled through and wrote about the greater part of Austria, visited this part of it, and he was so greatly struck with its appearance that he longed to make it his place of abode. His description of the spectacle which he beheld still holds good, and it may be thus rendered from the German:

"In Liburnia to the north there is a vast rampart against the wind; to the west and east there is, however, a beautiful mountain range, which is covered with all kinds of fruit-bearing trees, yielding the most exquisite fruit, such as figs, almonds, and olives, and all sorts of stone and other common fruits. Vines cling to and hang down from these trees. The garden hedges consist of tufts of pomegranates, laurels, and boxwood. All the foot-hills of the larger mountains are covered with fruit-bearing plants, and the low-roofed cottages of the peasants are scattered through these groves; there are fertile meadows higher up in the mountains where the finest sheep and goats find pasture. . . . To the south lies the open sea, which is studded with the most fertile islands; the water abounds with fish, and is covered with fishermen, who skim over it in their peculiar and specially constructed boats, and other light craft, which were famed for their swiftness even in the time of the Romans. The weather is mild all the year round; the air is clear, and fog is scarcely known."

Long before Balthasar Hacquet visited, described, and was enchanted with this beautiful region, it had attracted some Benedictine monks, who settled and built an abbey on the spot which is now known as Abbazia. They are supposed to have established themselves there so far back as the year 1300, but there are no entries in the archives at Fiume about their abbey till the year 1449. In 1453, Pope Nicholas the

Fifth issued a Bull authorising ecclesiastical penalties to be enforced against the evil-doers who did not pay tithes to the abbey, and who had appropriated ecclesiastical property. An inscription in the church, which has out-lasted the abbey, is as follows :

"1506, die 21 July, Symon Abbas fieri fecit," denoting that one Symon was the abbot at that time, and that the church had been restored by him. The particulars which have been preserved concerning the Benedictines at Abbazia largely relate to local disputes, and their interest is now purely professional and limited. Yet one of the incidents in a long-standing dispute between the Benedictines at Abbazia and the Augustines at Fiume is so curious, that it may be briefly told.

At the church festival on the 25th of July, 1579, the Vicar of Fiume presented himself as the delegate of his brethren there and claimed to open the dance. This pretension or pleasure being denied to him, he and the other visitors from Fiume withdrew from the festival. The result was that the inhabitants of Fiume ceased paying their annual visit to Abbazia in order to dance and make merry.

At the time of the Reformation many losses and changes befell this abbey. The Augustines of Fiume lost much property at Laibach, and, by way of compensation, the Benedictine abbey was annexed for ever to their monastery of San Giralmo. They sold the abbey to the Jesuits for 2,650 florins in 1723, and in 1735 the Jesuits sold it for 3,000 florins to Count John Ciculini. Fifteen years later the Jesuits obtained it again, and they kept it till 1773, when their order was dissolved. The revenue of the abbey was small; the building was neglected, and allowed to become a ruin; but the small church was preserved, and it still serves as the church of the people who dwell near it. It is a plain structure. An inscription states that it was last restored in 1792. As it is far too small to accommodate the congregation, many of whom cluster round the windows or sit outside the door, it may yet undergo a third transformation, and be rebuilt and enlarged.

Herr P. von Radics says, in the preface to a small work on Abbazia, that "Mother Nature had predestined that place to be a health resort." The intentions of Mother Nature may be excellent, yet something more is necessary before the place, which has countless charms, rises to the position for which it may be designed. The climate at Cannes is no finer now than it was before Lord Brougham accidentally visited it, built a house there, and brought it into notice. An inscription on a house in the East Bay at Mentone records that in 1855 the first discoverer of that spot as a health resort then arrived there; yet the fact of Dr. Henry Bennet going to Mentone for his health, practising as a physician during the winter, and writing a most fascinating book about it, must be numbered among the reasons why Mentone has increased and prospered. If our fleet had not frequently anchored in Torbay at the beginning of this century, and the delicate wives or children of the officers had not taken up their quarters on the coast there to await visits from their husbands or fathers, the balmy climate of Torquay might have never come into repute. Indeed, but half the task is accomplished after Nature has done her part. It is necessary, first, that a health resort should be rendered easily accessible, and secondly, that some one should appreciate its merits and make them known.

A wealthy inhabitant of Fiume, named Scarpa, is entitled to praise for discerning that the spot on which the Benedictines had settled was well fitted for others to regain health and enjoy life. Several years ago, he built the Villa Angiolina, close to the ruined abbey, and he laid out the gardens which surround the villa, filling them with rare plants, which would not flourish at Fiume in the open air, though that town is only a few miles distant. Moreover, he placed his villa at the disposal of the invalids among his acquaintance, and it gradually became known how much benefit could be derived by those in impaired health from a sojourn at Abbazia during the months when the weather at Fiume was trying and bleak. In 1860, the fame of Abbazia reached the ears of the Empress Maria Anna, and she spent some months in the Villa Angiolina. The King of Servia and several Austrian Archdukes have visited the place, and where Empresses and Kings and Archdukes take their pleasure, minor mortals are expected to congregate. In the case of Abbazia, this anticipation has been fully realised. During the winter season the available accommodation is barely sufficient to meet the demand.

Since the Villa Angiolina was built, and invalids began to visit Abbazia, the Southern Railway Company of Austria has bought land and built a large hotel there. The same company built the hotel at Toblach, in the Tyrol, where the lamented Emperor Frederick III. spent a few weeks during the last year of his life. That a railway company should build an hotel is natural enough; but that an hotel belonging to a railway company should be as well managed as one in private hands is almost unprecedented. The fact is that a few years ago the managing director of the Southern Railway decided that it would be an excellent speculation to attract persons to Abbazia, as by so doing he would bring grist to his mill in the form of passengers over his railway. Accordingly, land was bought, and an hotel was built there; this was called the Quarnero Hotel. A second, and larger one, called the Stephanie Hotel, was finished and opened three years ago, and now there are upwards of 200 rooms for the reception of visitors in the hotels, in two buildings adjoining them, and in the Villa Angiolina. Visitors can also find lodgings in several private houses. Abbazia is frequented in summer for sea bathing, the winter season beginning on the 15th of October and ending on the 15th of May, and the summer one on the 15th of May and ending on the 15th of October.

It is worthy of note that Abbazia is one of the very few places which offer to one class of invalids the attraction of a mild climate in winter, and to another that of excellent sea bathing in summer. There are many reasons why the best known places on the French and Italian Riviera should do likewise; yet custom or fashion has caused the beautiful spots from Cannes to Mentone, and from San Remo to Nervi, to be crowded with strangers during the winter months, and left to the inhabitants for the rest of the year.

The southern watering-places of England are resorted to all the year round, though the class visiting them during the winter season is a different one from that which can do so in the summer or autumn only. It is supposed that such a city as Nice would be intolerably hot in July and August, yet the heat during the day in these months is nearly as great at Hastings and Torquay. However, sixty thousand persons manage to exist at Nice during the summer. There, as at other spots on the Riviera, the mornings and evenings are cool and charming, and it is impossible to form a notion how enjoyable life is at any of them without paying a visit out of the season, when many of the hotels and shops are closed for lack of customers.

Several years ago, it was proposed to attract visitors to Nice during the summer; and with a view to effect this, an English company expended a large sum in building a pier on the model of the new pier at Brighton, with the addition of a restaurant at the end. Arrangements were made for sea bathing on a large scale and in great comfort, and it was believed that the experiment would prove successful in all respects. Shortly before the opening of the pier and restaurant, a fire destroyed everything except the iron pillars, which remained to demonstrate how well they were designed to withstand the shocks of wildest waves. It was said at the time that the fire was the work of an incendiary. The English company lost everything, and the ruined structure was long a blot on the prospect, and a reminder of wickedness or folly. A French company has been formed to complete the structure, so that Nice may yet have a summer season. At Abbazia, as at the places which I have named, the summer months are very hot; yet, so far as the experiment has been tried, the summer season at Abbazia has been a success.

Life at Abbazia in winter has some drawbacks which are not set forth in all the works which have been written about the place. In the winter of 1888, Sir Richard and Lady Burton spent three months in the Stephanie Hotel, and they communicated a narrative of their experiences to the *Vienna Weekly News*, a journal which for some years has represented the English Press in Austria-Hungary with great ability. As that journal is more widely circulated in Austria and Hungary than in England, the few extracts I shall make from its columns will be new to most of my readers. Some of Sir Richard's strictures appear to me a little too strong; but, then, he was in delicate health when at Abbazia, and the ailing are apt to be exacting. Moreover, he expected too much in looking for all the luxuries of Mecca within sight of Fiume, which he rather harshly styles "a one-horse harbour town." The natural beauties of the place charmed both Sir Richard and Lady Burton, and the few sentences in which they state their impression convey my own so accurately, that I shall quote them:

"The eastern shore of Istria offers in fine weather a charming panorama, and Abbazia lies at the head of the Fiume Gulf, which, for beauty and picturesqueness, ranks not much below the Bay of Naples. It is a noble basin, with outlines alternately *riant* and stern, gentle and majestic. Monte Maggiore, the culminating point of the little peninsula miscalled from the Danube, backs Abbazia with an altitude of 1,396 mètres, and the sea line of Croatia is subtended by the lofty Velebic, the Alp which connects the Julians of Carnia with the Dinarians of Dalmatia. To the south-east is the low-lying Island of Veglia, where, according to all experts, the sanatorium ought to have been built; further south the chine of Cherso, with its topping hummock, Monte Sys, acts as breakwater to the glorious natural harbour.

"The land, lying 2° north of Nice, will not produce the vegetation, tropical and sub-tropical, which glorifies southern France, yet the growth is characteristic, and contrasts sharply with that of the bleak uplands behind the shore. The thyme-laurel attains fine proportions, and 'lovrana' preserves the name *lauretum* (bay-grove) given to it by the Roman colonist. Magnolias, as in Southern Austria generally, reach a height of 25 ft. to 30 ft., and there is a single camphor tree, which flourishes despite all weathers. The arbutus bears its crimson berry and the mimosa its fluffy ball, while dracænas and yuccas, myrtles and lentisks, with here and there a standard bamboo and a fan palm, flourish by the side of firs and stone pines. We note also a Syrian harvest of pomegranates and chestnuts, olives and vines, set off, in the higher regions, by heath and gorse. The richness of the verdure and peculiarity of the growth marked the place in early days as rich in climatic advantages."

Sir Richard and Lady Burton did not find the winter climate so fine as they expected, the season being exceptional, as, indeed, they justly say, it generally is at health resorts where the chief industry is climate. Still, the winter of 1888 was really exceptional, as visitors to the French and Italian Rivieras had good reason to remember. They escaped the terrible bora, or north-west wind, which is the terror of Trieste, and they enjoyed some glorious days during December and January. They found the prevailing wind during the twelve weeks of the fashionable season to be the sirocco, which they did not like. That warm wind from Africa brings heavy showers in its train, being a wind which the late Charles Kingsley would have abhorred and denounced; but it is most grateful and soothing to the sensitive invalid, for whom a mild, moist air is as the breath of life.

As an experienced and most observant traveller, Sir Richard was careful to note the temperature during his stay, and he saw reason for doubting the correctness of some figures furnished by the correspondent of the *Lancet*, according to whom the mean temperature throughout the year is 56·4° Fahrenheit. He and his wife write that they carefully consulted every morning " the maximum and minimum thermometers of the little instrument box placed outside the Hôtel Stephanie, and on one occasion we found the mercury marking + for the night when ice, nearly an inch thick, stood within 100 yards. Consequently we determined that a pious fraud had been perpetrated on the thermometer and the foreigner." If this had occurred on several occasions, then I might have been disposed to concur in Sir Richard and Lady Burton's conclusion. It is quite possible, however, for the thermometer, which was not directly exposed to the air as was the water one hundred yards off, to register a higher temperature than it could have done if it had been placed where the process of freezing was in progress. The box containing the instruments is not well placed or arranged for accurately registering the extremes of heat and cold.

Dr. Szemere, in his work on "Abbazia as a Health

Resort," publishes the temperatures taken at seven o'clock in the morning during an entire year at Abbazia, Nice, Vienna, and Buda-Pesth, and copied from the Official reports of the Central Observatory at Vienna. These statistics may be regarded as absolutely trustworthy. On going through them I find that the temperature at Abbazia is given as being at freezing point on one morning, and on two mornings at a fraction above it, the days of the month on which this occurred being the 6th, 7th, and 8th of December. These figures were published before the Hôtel Stephanie was opened, and, as it is no secret that the thermometer sometimes registered a low temperature, it would be folly to attempt a fraud which, whether pious or the reverse, would assuredly be detected and ridiculed. Dr. Szemere gives the mean temperature for the year as 95° Fahrenheit in the sun, and 59° in the shade, and he puts the average winter temperature at from 42·8° to 44·6° Fahrenheit. Herr von Radics, on the other hand, puts it at from 44·6° to 46·4°.

Among the wants of this coast, the most conspicuous is the lack of running streams or springs of water. The few springs which exist are found near the shore, and the water in them is brackish. Great praise has been lavished upon Herr von Schüler for having erected a tank into which the water from several springs is pumped, and from which it is distributed throughout the hotels. Sir Richard Burton complains that when the sirocco blew, this water became brackish also; and he intimates that he was reduced to buy rain-water from the apothecary at Volosca. This is the simplest medicine which an apothecary ever supplied. As houses increase in number along this part of the coast—and, at the rate building is going on now, that increase will be rapid—the want of potable water will be the more keenly felt. The remedy is easy, and whoever applies it ought to reap profit from so doing. Let an establishment be erected for condensing the sea water on the Normandy principle, and let this water, when pumped up to a sufficient height and properly aërated, be supplied to the several houses.

The passages and principal rooms in the hotels and other buildings belonging to the railway company are lit with gas, candles being still used and charged for in the bedrooms. It is just as well that the antiquated practice of burning candles in the bedrooms has been continued, as few persons would have long survived the introduction of gas into them. The gas is not made from coal, but from coal tar, and no illuminant could be less satisfactory and more malodorous. There is always a difficulty in getting a light after the gas is turned on for the purpose.

The taps are opened to allow the air in the pipes to escape, and some are usually left open after the gas has begun to flow freely and before a light is applied. The result is to fill the passages with an odour which is inconceivably vile, and which causes one to fancy that all the drains had gone wrong at once. Why it did not occur to the authorities to introduce the electric light instead is the question which naturally occurs to one, but which it is easier to put than to answer. That the electric light will soon be introduced I have no doubt, and when this improvement is made, visitors will enjoy themselves more than they now do in the Hôtel Stephanie at nightfall.

Sir Richard and Lady Burton complain of the drains as well as the gas, and if their suffering from the drains was equal to that from the gas, I sincerely pity their hard lot. I should be wrong, however, in using the word drains to represent channels for carrying the sewage into the sea. The sea is not contaminated with foul and pestilent matter here, as it is at many of the places on the French Riviera, where typhoid fever and diphtheria are the consequences of improper drainage. Cesspools are the rule in Abbazia; but, owing to an error which it is impossible to excuse, they have been sunk, not outside the hotels, but within the inner court-yard. They are cleaned out once a month, and then for a day or two after this has taken place, the hotels become, to use the language of Sir Richard and Lady Burton, "fouler than the worst hospital of the pre-scientific age."

It is not my intention to repeat in detail all the objections which Sir Richard and Lady Burton have set forth in explicit and pointed terms. They will be found set forth at length in the numbers of the *Vienna Weekly News* for the 24th and 31st of July, and the 14th of August, 1888, and they were made because those in authority paid no heed to their complaints. The concluding sentences are that "Nature's materials are at Abbazia, but there is as yet no competency, no *savoir faire* to make use of them. And we do not recommend people to go there; in fact, we strongly dissuade them from so doing until the place is formed upon the principle that it ought to be, and, as we may add, it could be, by a mere turn of the wheel."

Unfortunately, perhaps, neither the drawbacks of bad smells nor of high charges hinder Austrians and Hungarians from filling the hotels at Abbazia. To them, indeed, the pestiferous odours have a familiar character—the hotels smell and remind them of home. After all, though the hotels belonging to the railway company are the largest, they are not the only buildings in Abbazia where visitors may find accommodation. If it be true, as Sir Richard and Lady Burton suggest, that the Island of Veglia would be a better site for a sanatorium, then a competing establishment may yet be erected there. If it be true, as I have been told by residents in Abbazia, that the climate at Volosca, which can be reached in twenty minutes in a carriage, has some advantages over that of Abbazia, then there is an opening for a competing hotel. The main fact is, that the climate of Abbazia and its vicinity is a pleasant one during the cold winter months; and when this is more widely known, the means for enjoying it will be amply supplied. I shall not be surprised if the railway company dispose of their hotels at Abbazia and confine their attention to developing their business in an appropriate fashion. The arrangements for conveying passengers are in great need of improvement, the trains being so timed as to start very early in the morning and very late at night. I may mention for the information of those who may desire to go to Abbazia, that direct trains run to the Mattuglie Station, on the Southern Railway, from Vienna, Prague, and Buda-Pesth, and that an hour's drive from this station brings the passenger to Abbazia. Trains from Venice or Trieste also carry passengers to Mattuglie Station, but carriages must be changed at least twice on the way. There is communication by sea, by road, and by rail with Fiume, the time occupied being two hours by rail and road, one hour by road alone, and an hour and a quarter by sea.

The result of long observations on this part of the coast shows that the winter lasts three months, from the beginning of December to the end of February; the spring two, from the beginning of March to the end of April; the summer five, from the beginning of May to the end of September, the months of October and November being the autumn. Those who go for sea bathing in the summer, if ailing, are expected to pursue the treatment under medical advice. They are put on a regular course of diet, and the "cure" is pursued as systematically as at Carlsbad or any other Austrian health resort. During winter, the "cure" can be continued within doors. A large bath-house contains all sorts of baths, including electric baths, which Sir Richard Burton styles "expensive humbugs." The hot sea baths are most in request; and, as Dr. Szemere affirms, many persons suffering from general debility, or from irritability of the chest, may be greatly benefited by the hot sea baths and mild climate of Abbazia during the winter months.

The majority visit Abbazia to escape from the cold of Trieste or Vienna, Prague or Buda-Pesth, and other cities in Austria and Hungary. Both those who are well, and those who are ailing, must be as surprised as Sir Richard Burton was at the absence of an apothecary's shop in Abbazia. As a rule, no health resort is supposed to be complete without an apothecary's shop. What is the use, indeed, of a physician writing a prescription if the patient cannot get it made up? Sir Richard and Lady Burton pathetically write that, as it is twenty minutes' drive to Volosca, where an apothecary dispenses medicines, "an unfortunate in the hotel at Abbazia suddenly taken ill during the night might easily slip out of the world before the necessary drug could be procured." They lay the blame upon the directors of the railway company, who ask an exorbitant rent, and thus deny an apothecary the chance of making profit by setting up shop. On the other hand, visitors are consoled with the intimation that a small stock of medicine is kept in the hotel for their use in case of necessity.

The last sentences which I shall extract from the lively epistles of Sir Richard and Lady Burton relate to the natives of the place. They are chiefly Croats; the priest preaches in Slav, and during the service " the people howl (we cannot use any other word) a hymn in Slav, which appears to be of about ten bars in length and *da capo*, till your head is ready to burst;

they never change either words or tune." Again, they write of these Croats:

"If, unhappily, you address a Croatian peasant in Italian, he either turns his back upon you with a growl, or follows your retreating form with hateful eyes. These half-reclaimed races not only hate all strangers, they abhor every one but themselves, and they have opprobrious words to denote all but their own caste. If an Italian, the foreigner is called *Taljancic*, or *polenta*, or *irredenta*; if a German, he becomes *nemcur*, or *nemckutar*, or *krödel*; if a Hungarian, he is *Magyaron*, or *padella*, or *paprika*, the last from the national condiment. But *en revanche* these churls are honest and harmless, and women and children may walk about the nooks and corners unprotected, which is more than we can say for our English cross-country by-ways."

There are few amusements at Abbazia. The band of a Hungarian regiment comes twice a week from Fiume and plays in the open air when the weather is fine. Many excursions can be made to places of historical interest, and there are several beautiful walks. The Austrian Tourists' Club of Vienna has rendered Abbazia the service, in common with many other places, of keeping the old walks in order, of forming new ones, and of placing seats at points where the view is most striking. I think it probable that the place will continue to grow in importance and popularity. The seekers after change will find it here. They will enjoy lovely scenery, fine air, and the excellent wines of the country. To many, the good wines will not be the least among the attractions. The greatest treat which a peasant can have is a glass of the sweet Malmsey, which is one of the dessert wines produced here; but the other wines, for which the peasants care less, will better please the palates of the more fastidious. Both English and American visitors to Abbazia will have the satisfaction of traversing a most interesting part of Europe when journeying to it, and of finding, when they arrive, that they have reached a charming place of which few of their countrymen have even heard and still fewer have ever seen.

CHAPTER XV.

GORIZIA.

When Byron dedicated his tragedy of *Marino Faliero* to Goethe, he wrote: "You have been fortunate, sir, not only in the writings which have illustrated your name, but in the name itself, it being sufficiently musical for the articulation of posterity. In this you have the advantage of some of your countrymen, whose names would perhaps be immortal also if anybody could pronounce them." It is doubtful whether the English poet could correctly pronounce the name of his great German contemporary; and it is certain that nobody now pronounces Byron's own name as he and his schoolfellows did, which was in the manner that the name would be pronounced by a Frenchman. It is with a view to render the pronunciation easier to English readers that I have chosen the Italian form of spelling the chief city of the county of Görz and Gradisca, of which I am about to give an account. The inhabitants of that small and picturesque city are Germans, Italians, and Slavs, and they name it after their own fashion, the first calling it Görz, the second Gorizia, and the third Gorica. Though the German form is that used in railway time tables, yet, as Italian is the language which is generally spoken in the place and neighbourhood, Gorizia is the name most frequently heard, and if not the most accurate, it is at least the most familiar. Moreover, it has the advantage of being uttered very easily by foreign lips.

The Emperor of Austria and King of Hungary numbers among his many minor titles that of Count of Görz and Gradisca. Gorizia is the capital of this county, which extends over fifty-three and a half square miles, and is bounded on the west by Venetia, on the north by Carinthia, on the east by Krain, and on the south by Istria, by the district in which lies the city of Trieste, and by the Adriatic. Trieste is reached in two hours by rail, and the Italian frontier at Cormons in twenty minutes. The first building erected was the castle which still towers above the city; the earliest houses clustered for protection under the shadow of the ramparts and on the slope below them. In the year 1307, the inhabitants received the privilege accorded to dwellers in a borough. How long before that date the castle was built is not accurately known, the first mention of it being in the year 1000. Other houses were built below those on the castle slope, a moat and wall were carried round their unprotected sides, and such was the beginning of the city of Gorizia.

The place prospered from the outset, the site being a pleasant one and suited for settlement. It had its trials, however, one of the most severe being an earthquake in 1348, and others being attacks from the Venetians, who captured the city and retained possession of it during twelve months. The citizens were not only attached to Gorizia, but they were proud of the laws for its government, which were framed in the fourteenth century, and of which a printed copy is still extant. The first church, which is now the cathedral, was built in 1400; a Minorite monastery was built some time before, and a Capuchin monastery some time afterwards. The fine climate of Gorizia has rendered the place attractive to religious orders. In 1615, the Jesuits arrived and established a training college, which was largely attended, and they built the church of Ignatius, which is now the most conspicuous object in the centre of the city. Their college was turned into a barrack, and all their property was confiscated by the Austrian Government in 1773.

For two centuries before this event, the county

of Gorizia had belonged to the House of Austria, the family of the Counts of that name having become extinct. Up to the sixteenth century, the population was chiefly German; but, owing to repeated wars with Venice, the interruption of communication with Germany, and the immigration from Italy, the Italian element became the leading one. The city continued to flourish. In 1576, Count Porzia, the Papal Nuncio, wrote that Gorizia was a place "where much business is transacted, and where one can buy linen and cloth." He also wrote that "the people are German in their food, drinking, and their apparel, and that three tongues are commonly spoken, German, Slavonic, and Italian." But, while the manners were those of Germany, the race was Italian, and the Germans proper then appeared as a small colony in a city of Italy.

At the beginning of the eighteenth century another change occurred, and both the Emperor Charles the Sixth and the Empress Maria Theresa did their utmost to Germanise Gorizia, making a knowledge of the German tongue indispensable for obtaining a post under Government. An Archbishopric of Gorizia was founded by the Empress. This region suffered during the cruel and bloody wars which the first French Republic began for the promotion of fraternity and for the regeneration of mankind, and which Bonaparte prosecuted for his own aggrandisement and glory. The county of Görz and Gradisca was separated by him from Austria, incorporated with the Kingdom of Illyria, and united to France. This union lasted from 1809 till 1814. In the latter year the county was restored to Austria. In 1861, the Emperor Francis Joseph the First decreed that the county of Görz and Gradisca should be constituted a Crownland, with a Parliament for the regulation of its local affairs. Since then the history of the city has been uneventful. The city has continued to flourish, and of late years it has numbered among its industries the modern one of profiting by the strangers who select it as a place of sojourn on account of the excellence of its climate. It is as a health resort that Gorizia is probably destined to play as useful a part as any of which its history bears record.

Baron von Czoernig, the author of a most elaborate work on the history of Gorizia, has styled it the "Austrian Nice." Dr. Schatzmayer, a physician practising at Trieste, who has visited Gorizia more than forty times, who has done so for the sake of his own health, who has sent patients there, and has written a small work on the place and its climate, is not quite able to agree with Baron von Czoernig, and he says that Gorizia is emphatically the Nice of

Austria and not that of France. The case resembles that of Klopstock being hailed as the German Milton—"a very German Milton" was the unwelcome, but not inappropriate comment of Coleridge. According to Dr. Schatzmayer, this place is one of the best Sub-Alpine health resorts. It is much less known than most of them, where visitors from England and America as well as the European Continent abound, the number of Englishmen and Americans being small to whom Gorizia is a familiar name.

The situation of Gorizia is most beautiful, being at the upper end of a valley, fifteen miles long and seven miles and a half wide, through which the river Isonzo flows. The water of this river is the colour of turquoise. The whole plain is under cultivation; fruit-bearing trees predominate; vines cling to the trees and hang down between them. An excellent wine is made from the grapes. Olive and fig trees are plentiful, and there are so many evergreens that the plain is seldom quite naked and leafless, even in the dead of winter. It is not uncommon for apple and pear trees to produce ripe fruit twice within twelve months. The geological formation is sandstone, and the porous soil rapidly absorbs the rain. Two hours after the heaviest downpour the roads are almost dry. Visitors from the North are astounded to see the streets being watered in the month of January.

Protected on three sides from cold winds by wooded mountains and open towards the south, there is a general resemblance between the situation of Gorizia and that of Arco, near the top of Lake Garda. Dr. Schatzmayer says that the winter climate of Gorizia is similar to the spring climate of Mid-Germany. The temperature is almost the same as that of Venice, and only about 3° Fahrenheit lower than that of Rome in winter.

Dr. Schatzmayer honestly admits that the winter climate of Gorizia is different from that of Madeira, Cairo, Palermo, and Mentone; he contends, however, that it has some advantages which are not to be found at any of these places. One is the combination of inland Alpine air with the air of the sea, the distance from the Adriatic not being too great to hinder the influence of the sea being felt. Another is the moderate range of the temperature, the consequence being that there is less liability to chill or catarrh at Gorizia than at places where the variation is greater. Snow is rarely seen except on the distant mountain peaks; fogs are uncommon, and, though rain often falls, the days are few in number during which it falls without ceasing. The half, or at least the third, of each winter's day is generally bright and clear.

As contrasted with Nice and Mentone, the stillness of the air at Gorizia is remarkable, the surrounding mountains sheltering it from violent winds. For an invalid a clear sky, warm sunshine, and the absence of wind are most desirable, and Gorizia is favoured in these essentials to the enjoyment of life and for the recovery of health. The houses have a marked advantage in one respect over those on the French and Italian Riviera. At Gorizia perpetual sunshine is not counted upon by the inhabitants, nor is it the rule at the health resorts in southern France and Italy. Yet the inhabitants of the towns on the Riviera of Italy and France seem to think it unnecessary to make provision against gloomy and cold days. They require so little artificial heat when the sun shines brightly that they are unprepared for the days when the sky is overcast and the cold is intense. On such days an invalid, and even a person in good health, shivers and shakes, and longs to be near a blazing hot fire, or for the heat of a well-made stove. The fires which are lit in rooms of the houses from Cannes to Spezia are bright and illusory; they cost much and are worth little, giving forth an abundance of smoke and scarcely any warmth. The rooms at Gorizia are provided with excellent porcelain stoves, and when it is cold out of doors the passages and rooms within are warm and comfortable. There is nothing Italian in the arrangements for heating the houses.

Since my visit to Gorizia and the appearance of my

account in *The Times,* an Englishman, who has lived there for some time, has contributed a description of the place and its people to the *Vienna Weekly News.* The testimony of a stranger, who has had ample opportunity for learning the drawbacks and advantage of a foreign city, being more valuable than that of one whose visit to it may be too short to entitle him to speak with authority, I extract the following passage from this gentleman's account, which relates to the important and interesting subject of climate: "The climate of Gorizia is half sea and half mountain climate. The air is particularly pure—dry, yet not too dry— mountain air tempered by sea air. Many invalids cannot stand the sea air of Nice. Many invalids cannot stand the mountain air of St. Moritz or Meran. The air of Gorizia is a happy medium. Invalids are sent from Nice to Montreux. The climate of Gorizia, while possessing the properties of the climate of Montreux, is very much milder. Gorizia is decidedly milder than Meran, though, as a rule, very far from so mild as Nice. . . . Gorizia is a favourite winter resort with old men who are forced to study climatic conditions; also of men who, though not old, are no longer young, whom *force majeure* has compelled to relinquish the pomps and vanities of a wicked world. One would never come to Gorizia to seek gaiety or society. But it is by no means only the hipped, the hypochondriac, or invalid who select Gorizia as a winter resort or place of abode. Nor is it that there is not 'society' in Gorizia. Quite the contrary. The society is good, but 'society' does not go into, or 'go in for' society. As we talk in England of three middle classes, the upper, middle, and lower, so might we talk here of three aristocratic classes, the upper, middle, and lower, the distinctions between them are as scrupulously absurd, and as clearly marked in the one case as in the other. . . .

"The houses in Gorizia are infinitely preferable to the houses of Nice or Naples, all having double windows and stoves. One can keep oneself warm here indoors, when the weather is severe—more than can be said for many of the houses of Naples and Nice. . . . Cold winds, stone floors, fireless rooms are more trying to the invalid than even frost and snow, with calm days, carpets, and fireplaces. One of the distinctive features of the climate of Gorizia is the general absence of windy days. To one who has felt and suffered from the well-nigh daily chilly blast, which during spring sweeps across Florence, to one who has experienced the 'mistrale' of Nice, or even to one who has had to close the lips before the crisp, keen sea breezes of the Bay of Naples, to such, this advantage will be appreciable. The Meran doctors order their patients to go out in rain, snow, and fog, but not in wind. Such an occurrence as a fog or mist at Gorizia, is as rare as snow at Nice. Snow rarely falls at Gorizia, and never lies. We rarely see it on the tops of our nearest hills."

What strikes the visitor nearly as much as the fine scenery around Gorizia is the scrupulous cleanliness of the city. Few Southern cities are kept in better order, as even the narrow lanes in the older part, where the houses are crowded together, are free from noisome smells and unpleasant sights. To hear so much Italian spoken in streets so clean is a novelty. The water supply is excellent, the water being brought from springs at a distance. Great care is taken to prevent the soil in the neighbourhood from being contaminated with sewage. The streets and houses are lighted with gas, and the gasworks are less hideous in appearance than those in other places, the entrance to them being covered with creeping plants, and trees surrounding them. The public garden, which dates from 1861, is one of the city's attractions. It is well laid out and kept; the terrace, looking towards the south and sheltered behind, forms the favourite spot whereon to rest or walk in winter. As growth is never entirely suspended, some plants are always in leaf or coming into flower in the garden.

In the fields, the grain chiefly cultivated is maize,

which forms a large part of the people's food; vegetables such as peas, asparagus, and broccoli are largely grown. Many beehives are to be seen near the peasants' houses. The fruit of Gorizia forms an important article of export; in its dried form it is sent all over the Continent. The kinds which are most abundant and in request include cherries and grapes, apples and pears, plums and apricots, peaches and figs, almonds and chestnuts. As the quantity exported yields as much as £40,000, it will be seen that fruit-growing is conducted on a very large scale.

Many a larger place than Gorizia cannot boast, as it may do, of possessing a public library. It was founded in 1823. The volumes are upwards of 20,000 in number, and they are not only accessible to the public daily, but they can also, under certain conditions, be taken away for reading at home.

Since these two sentences about the library were written its existence has been called in question. I first learned about the library from Dr. Schatzmayer's small work on Gorizia; when there I was shown the library itself, and yet in an article in the *Corriere de Gorizia*, commenting on what I had written, it is stated as an error of mine that Gorizia "possesses a public library of 20,000 volumes, founded in 1823," and the question is asked, "Where is this library?" Journalists are often reproached with professing to be omniscient; the conductors of the *Corriere de Gorizia* are free from that failing. They seem to me to be open to the reproach of knowing too little. They might profit by a visit to the library in their own city, which, as I can affirm on the written authority of the Librarian, Professor Dr. Baar, actually contains 22,403 volumes, and 3,982 works in parts and sheets.

The English resident from whose articles I have already quoted, gives a detailed account of the amusements at Gorizia, and I now substitute his version for that which I gave in *The Times:*

"At the end of the Corso we pass the theatre, a pretty and comfortable little house, with stalls, pit, and gallery, and the rest of the space devoted to tiers of private boxes. The highest price for a private box is five shillings! We have an autumn, winter (Carnival), and spring (Easter) theatrical season —generally, companies *en voyage* for larger centres, which take in Gorizia *en route*. The Gorizian has a high standard of merit; a Gorizian audience is rather exacting—considering the price paid for the play. And the Gorizians are ambitious. They have had Ristori and Patti here, and now they wish Sarah Bernhardt! They had a season of Italian Opera all to themselves last Easter, bringing a special company from Milan. Yet theatrical companies have a hard time of it here. If an Italian Company comes, the

Germans won't patronise it, and when a German Company comes it generally comes to grief, as 'the Italians'—the Italian speaking party—won't patronise it.

"There is also a summer theatre, situated in a neat little garden, attached to one of the hotels. Here we have smoked our cigar, and drunk our beer, listening to Italian Opera performed by not at all a bad scratch company of artists. Yet, strange to say, this form of entertainment, which in London would draw an over-crowded garden, does not meet with the support of the people here, who, however, old or young, high or low, will scramble for places at a performance of the Marionettes.

"In the same building as the Winter Theatre are the Club Rooms of the *Societa Cura Climatica*. This is the *Curhaus* of Gorizia. There is a reading-room, tolerably well supplied with newspapers, the *Graphic* being the only English print honoured with a place on the tables. Entertainments of one kind or other are given weekly. A dance is an event of rare occurrence in the *Curhaus*. The principal dances are given in the Clubs during Carnival season. A private dance is almost 'an unknown quantity' in Gorizia."

The visitor will probably think that the hotel accommodation might be improved. When I arrived,

I asked a native of the place, holding an official position, which was the best hotel, and he told me the question was one which it was difficult to answer. There are five or six hotels, and they are much the same in all respects except situation. They are not uncomfortable from an Italian or German point of view. Indeed, they are quite as good as those in any city of Italy or Germany of the same size. Yet English and American travellers, and invalids in particular, would prefer to inhabit hotels upon a more modern plan than those of Gorizia. The palace of Baron Formentini, built in 1863, and standing amid beautiful grounds, has been converted into a boarding-house, and is much frequented by winter visitors. I know nothing of its merits as a place of sojourn, but I have admired the house and its site. There are many villas which are built on a modern plan, and in which the visitor can find more comfortable accommodation than in the hotels.

Dr. Schatzmayer remarks that most articles of food are as dear at Gorizia as at Trieste, but that, as they are less adulterated, they are much more nourishing. He praises the honesty of the people, saying that thieving is very rare, and that the air of Gorizia is pure in all respects. Mr. Vervega, a banker here, who, though not a native, has lived long enough to understand the place thoroughly, confirms from his personal experience all that I had read in favour of it. As he knows both England and America as well as his native Austria, his opinion is the better worth having. Last year, Mr. Vervega contributed an article on Gorizia to the *Vienna Weekly News,* and the following short extract from what he has written may be better worth reproducing than the tenor of his conversation with me:

"You will find here, so far as climate goes, all that you can get at the Riviera or the Engadine. In summer you can 'lay off' in the shade and enjoy lovely nights, and, what is more, your purse will not empty so soon, for what you spend in three months elsewhere and get scanty value for, you can thrive here upon for six months and have plenty and good. Come, let me take you to the market-place—Piazza dell' Erbe! Listen to the sound of voices and laughter! Yes—you do hear German and Slavonic, but the native tongue, the Italian, is dominant; and what surprises me is, those very ultra-Germans and Slavs are doing their best to pass off as Italians, or rather natives. Inspect the variety of vegetables offered to you. Fancy yourself in your native northern home, in mid-winter, and what you pay its weight in gold for elsewhere, here in Friuli, particularly in Gorizia, you have, so to say, for half nothing. In spring and summer you are puzzled to select from the variety of fruits or vegetables—melons, peaches, grapes, plums, etc. But where does all this come from? And what of the thousands of hampers and baskets full of the soil's produce sent daily by rail to the very north of Europe, and yet plenty left for the use of the townspeople? Your cook cannot complain of the butchers; prime beef and veal is at the most 8d. a pound, poultry is also very cheap, spring chickens about 6d. a pair;* the fish market every Friday and fast day is fully supplied from the Adriatic, two hours from here, with such a variety of fish that you fancy yourself at the fish market of Algiers. Lastly, your butler can fill your cellar with sound, pure, native red or white wine at 2½d. per pint. Butter, milk, and all the necessaries of life are at the same cheap rate. Are not these matters and figures worth taking into consideration nowadays? Your gold currency gains about 25 per cent., a very important matter in liquidating yearly accounts. Thus, from an economical point of view, paterfamilias can do the Continent by spending a winter or summer in Gorizia, much more at his ease than elsewhere, as, for instance, Belgium, the Rhine, Switzerland, and so on."

It is with reluctance, if not regret, that I give Mr. Vervega's testimony concerning the cheapness

---

* Mr. Vervega informs me that poultry is bought at Gorizia with the intention of fattening it for the table.

of living here. I can affirm, from personal experience, that the hotel prices are half those which I paid at Abbazia, and much less than those at the best-known health resorts. Let it be generally known that Gorizia is a cheap as well as a pleasant place to live in, and it will not long remain either cheap or pleasant. Many of my countrymen, and still more of my countrywomen, are constantly on the look-out for some spot where they can go and economise, and several places have been spoilt by the influx of those who expect to get all the luxuries of existence for a trifling sum. After all, a place where living is as cheap as in Gorizia has its drawbacks, and, as I have hinted, the hotels are rather too Continental in their arrangements to satisfy fastidious English and Americans, who, if they desire home comforts, must pay as dearly for them at Gorizia as at any other place on the European Continent. When the hotels are as fine as those on the Riviera, on the Rhine, and in Switzerland, the prices will be in keeping, that is, equal to those of London, Paris, and even New York.

Many languages are spoken in Gorizia. The visitor who does not speak Italian or German will regret having taken up his abode there. That curious linguistic compound which so many persons in England

and America, of whom the majority are women, call and consider to be "French," will prove of no service in Gorizia. This French bears the same relation to the language of France that the Pigeon English of Hongkong or Shanghai does to the English of England and America. I have met with many persons who avowed their capacity for speaking "French" fluently, but I have seldom met with any one who understood all the words which they uttered with an accent as strange as the words. This "French" is the modern equivalent to the unknown tongue of Holy Writ. Yet even those who speak good French would not find it much easier to get on in Gorizia than those who speak English only.

A few years ago, a large number of Frenchmen visited Gorizia, and were present at the burial there of the last of the French Bourbons. In addition to the other things which make this place noteworthy may be cited the fact that the Count de Chambord passed the last year of his life and is entombed in Gorizia. Three years ago, his wife was laid beside him. Charles the Tenth of France had been carried in 1836 to his last resting-place in the same vault. This vault lies under the high altar of the church belonging to the Franciscan monastery of Castagnavizza. The monastery is perched on an eminence immediately outside the city, and the view from it is second only to that from the castle, which rises at a short distance in front. In a beautiful passage, which makes the reader feel that prose is sometimes scarcely less poetical than verse, Macaulay dilates on the vanity of human hopes and human destiny in relation to St. Peter's Chapel in the Tower of London. A lesson quite as sad and impressive is taught by the spectacle of the tombs of the Bourbons at Castagnavizza. Charles the Tenth ascended the throne after having tasted the bitterness of exile. If he had profited in the slightest degree by experience, had possessed a little tact and even a small portion of common-sense, he would have retained the crown of France, would have died to the great grief of his subjects, and been buried with pomp in the grand cathedral of St. Denis. As it was, he became an exile and a wanderer for the second time, found an asylum again in Holyrood House, and, when nearing his end and longing for sunnier skies than those which shroud "the gray Metropolis of the North," he arrived at Gorizia on October 25, and died there on November 6, 1836.

In the same vault where his coffin was laid were afterwards placed those of the Duke and Duchess of Angoulême. There, in 1883, the coffin of the Count de Chambord was also deposited, and that of his wife was placed alongside it three years ago. The Count de Chambord was once on the verge of being hailed by the French as Henry the Fifth, but he emphatically declined to make the trivial concession which was first required of him. There is nothing on the coffin of Charles the Tenth to show that he had worn the crown of France, while a small gilt crown on that of the Count de Chambord represents the crown which was never put upon his head. In this narrow vault lie entombed more than the remains of a few members of the House of Bourbon. In the coffin surmounted with a crown are enclosed the hopes of many millions of Frenchmen, and the aspirations of a dynasty to which France owes much of her glory, and to which she may attribute no small portion of her trials and misfortunes.

When emerging from this dismal vault and seeing the bright sky and sweet sunshine again, the beauty of the prospect banishes all sombre thoughts. Every place is alike when the last hour strikes; and, though the cry of the ancient Greek was to die in the sunlight, yet the closing scene must be the same to the expiring mortal, whether the place be lovely or wretched, whether the sky be dark or bright. A beholder of the scene from the terrace outside of the church at Castagnavizza may forget for the moment the inevitable end. While his eyes are turned towards the exquisite spectacle, the uppermost thought in his mind must be that Gorizia is a beautiful spot to live in.

THE END.

www.ingramcontent.com/pod-product-compliance
Lightning Source LLC
Chambersburg PA
CBHW030002240426
43672CB00007B/795